S0-AZA-235

H. L. Haas G. Buzsàki (Eds.)

Synaptic Plasticity in the Hippocampus

Foreword by E. Grastyan

With 55 Figures and 3 Tables

Springer-Verlag Berlin Heidelberg New York
London Paris Tokyo

Professor Helmut L. Haas, M.D.
II. Physiologisches Institut
Johannes Gutenberg-Universität
Saarstrasse 21, 6500 Mainz
Federal Republic of Germany

Professor György Buzsàki, M.D.
Department of Neurosciences MO24
University of California at San Diego
La Jolla, CA 92093, USA

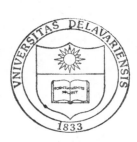

QP
383
.25
.596
1988

ISBN 3-540-18599-2 Springer-Verlag Berlin Heidelberg New York
ISBN 0-387-18599-2 Springer-Verlag New York Berlin Heidelberg

This work is subject to copyright. All rights are reserved, whether the whole or part of the material is concerned, specifically the rights of translation, reprinting, re-use of illustrations, recitation, broadcasting, reproduction on microfilms or in other ways, and storage in data banks. Duplication of this publication or parts thereof is only permitted under the provisions of the German Copyright Law of September 9, 1965, in its version of June 24, 1985, and a copyright fee must always be paid. Violations fall under the prosecution act of the German Copyright Law.

© Springer-Verlag Berlin Heidelberg 1988
Printed in Germany

The use of general descriptive names, trade names, trade marks, etc. in this publication, even if the former are not especially identified, is not to be taken as a sign that such names, as understood by the Trade Marks and Merchandise Marks Act, may accordingly be used freely by anyone.

Product Liability: The publisher can give no guarantee for information about drug dosage and application thereof contained in this book. In every individual case the respective user must check its accuracy by consulting other pharmaceutical literature.

Offsetprinting: Druckhaus Beltz, Hemsbach/Bergstr.
Binding: J. Schäffer GmbH & Co. KG, Grünstadt
2125/3145-543210

Foreword

This is the second time that I have had the honor of opening an international symposium dedicated to the functions of the hippocampus here in Pècs. It was a pleasure to greet the participants in the hope that their valuable contributions will make this meeting a tradition in this town.

As one of the hosts of the symposium, I had the sorrowful duty to remind you of the absence of a dear colleague, Professor Graham Goddard. His tragic and untimely death represents the irreparable loss of both a friend and an excellent researcher. This symposium is dedicated to his memory.

If I compare the topics of the lectures of this symposium with those of the previous one, a striking difference becomes apparent. A dominating tendency of the previous symposium was to attempt to define hippocampal function or to offer data relevant to supporting or rejecting existing theoretical positions. No such tendency is reflected in the titles of the present symposium, in which most of the contributions deal with hippocampal phenomena at the most elementary level. Electrical, biochemical, biophysical, and pharmacological events at the synaptic, membrane, or intracellular level are analyzed without raising the question of what kind of integral functions these elementary phenomena are a part of. What might be the cause of this theoretical indifference? Perhaps disappointment with the inefficiency of the theoretical debates of more than three decades? Or the recognition that our knowledge of intrahippocampal information processing is still inadequate for verification of functional theories? Most of the theoreticians, faithfully following the traditions of functional localization were looking for a single, exclusive function, like orienting, attention, internal inhibition, spatial mapping, working memory, etc. The feasibility of such an approach would now be questioned by many. Though highly simplistic, it is tempting to make the assumption that the unique macroscopic shape of the hippocampus, resembling a seahorse, or its orderly inner organization, resembling random access memory, might have been suggestive of an exclusive and unitary function. In the course of my own speculations about hippocampal function, whenever a plausible hypothesis emerged I could not banish from my mind the embarrassing clinical evidence that humans with a complete inborn absence of the hippocampal formation do not show any lack of the capacities attributed to the hippocampus. If the function attributed to the hippocampus presupposes its unique morphological organization and connections, one can wonder how this peculiar function could be replaced by brain structures with completely different organization and connections.

These serious uncertainties are sufficient for me to accept the pursuit suggested by the titles of the present symposium as a new and promising strategy. It seems reasonable and compelling to get closer to elementary hippocampal processes by putting aside our preconceptions suggested by existing theories. This approach is also justified by the spectacular developments of electrophysiological, biochemical, and biophysical techniques. It is, however, conceivable that investigations with these highly refined techniques will uncover basic and universal processes of neural plasticity rather than information on hippocampal functions. In this context, because of its relatively simple organization, the hippocampus is undoubtedly one of the most promising targets among brain structures. Insights gained concerning the basic processes of plasticity would be a formidable achievement even if they do not add anything special to understanding the function of the hippocampus itself. We cannot however exclude the possibility that investigations with these advanced methods might also uncover hippocampal mechanisms allowing the formulation of an entirely new hypothesis about its function which has remained hidden so far just because of our traditional preconceptions.

Pècs, August 13, 1987   Endre Grastyan

Preface

This volume contains the papers presented at a satellite symposium on synaptic plasticity in the hippocampus, held at Pècs, Hungary, on 13–15 August, 1987, preceding the International Brain Research Organisation (IBRO) Congress in Budapest. The emblem of this symposium, as depicted on the cover of this volume, was the triton, a winged hippocampus, the wings signifying plasticity.

The meeting was dedicated to Graham Goddard, who had agreed to participate before his untimely death in a hiking accident in New Zealand on 15 January 1987. T.V.P. Bliss gave an account on his life and personality.

Like the meeting, this book provides a comprehensive survey of the rapidly growing field of hippocampal plasticity. The last decade has generated a multitude of studies using in vitro model systems to examine long-lasting changes at the synaptic level. At the same time, considerable concern continues to be expressed regarding the significance of in vitro findings for in vivo adaptive and maladaptive changes, such as memory and epilepsy. Problems in interpreting the results of different approaches and methods in the study of synaptic plasticity in the hippocampus were discussed by researchers from various disciplines: morphology, biochemistry, neurology, psychology, pharmacology, electrophysiology and molecular biology. Accordingly, the book is divided into seven parts, focussing on problems of synaptic, transmitter, and molecular mechanisms of long-term potentiation (LTP); control of hippocampal excitability, kindling and epilepsy; the LTP model; and physiological plasticity.

We are indebted to the *Fonds für versuchstierfreie Forschung,* Zürich; Boehringer, Ingelheim, F.R.G.; Upjohn, U.S.A.; Smith Kline & French, U.K., and several local Hungarian firms whose sponsorship made the symposium possible. Special thanks are extended to Gisela Günther, Mainz, and Zsuzsa Herzfeld, Pècs, who provided invaluable help with the preparation of the meeting and the volume.

January, 1988

Helmut L. Haas, Mainz
György Buzsàki, San Diego

Table of Contents

Synaptic Mechanisms of Long-Term Potentiation

Transmitter Mechanisms of Long-Term Potentiation

What Does Long-Term Potentiation Model?

Molecular Mechanisms of Long-Term Potentiation

Control of Excitability in Hippocampus

Kindling and Epilepsy

Physiological Plasticity

List of Contributors*

Abraham, W.C.   3, 35, 122[1]
Akase, E.   198
Al-Ani, N.   38
Albert, K.   109
Andersen, P.   109
Anderson, W.W.   180
Anwyl, R.   144
Avoli, M.   9
Baimbridge, K.G.   169
Balzer, J.R.   190
Berger, T.W.   190
Bergis, O.   208
Bilkey, D.K.   3
Blake, J.F.   38
Bliss, T.V.P.   42, 45, 110
Bloch, V.   208
Bonhaus, D.W.   70
Bramham, C.R.   205
Brown, M.W.   38, 146, 194
ten Bruggencate, G.   159
Burge, B.C.   70
Buzsàki, G.   VII, 45, 90
Cairns, N.J.   146
Campiche, P.   155
Chirwa, S.S.   102
Clements, M.P.   110
Cline, H.T.   17
Coan, E.J.   38, 73
Collingridge, G.L.   31, 38, 73
Czopf, J.   45
Desmond, N.L.   93
Diamond, D.M.   96

Disterhoft, J.F.   198
Doyere, V.   208
Drapeau, C.   9
Dunwiddie, T.V.   96
Errington, M.L.   42, 110
Frey, U.   126
Frotscher, M.   87
Goddard, G.V.   3, 122
Grastyan, E.   V
Gray, R.   57
Greene, R.W.   77
Greengard, P.   109
Haas, H.L.   VII, 42, 77, 90
Halgren, E.   202
Hamon, B.   6
Harty, T.P.   190
Hashimoto, T.   81
Heimrich, B.   77
Heinemann, U.   6, 184
Heit, G.   202
Herron, C.E.   31
Higashima, M.   24
Hirotsu, I.   81
Hopf, A.   163
Hopkins, H.F.   57
Horikawa, Y.   81
Horváth, Z.   45
Hu, G.-Y.   109
Hvalby, Ø.   109
Ibata, Y.   81
Ishihara, T.   81
Ito, K.   46

---

*The address of the authors is given on the first page of each contribution
[1]Page, on which contribution commences

Synaptic Mechanisms
of Long-Term Potentiation

Long-Term Potentiation of Feed-Forward Inhibition in Hippocampus: Extracellular Evidence

G. V. GODDARD, E. W. KAIRISS, W. C. ABRAHAM, and D. K. BILKEY

Department of Psychology and The Neuroscience Centre, University of Otago, Box 56, Dunedin, New Zealand

A decrease in the slope of the EPSP-spike (E-S) relationship accompanies long-term potentiation (LTP) of the perforant path input to the dentate gyrus in normal, but not picrotoxin treated animals. When granule cell LTP is reduced by concurrent commissural tetanisation, a decrease in spike height and a shift to the right of the E-S curve is observed. Finally, short latency, low threshold units show a reduced firing threshold following perforant path tetanisation. These data are consistent with the hypothesis that LTP occurs at perforant path synapses onto feed-forward inhibitory interneurones.

Tetanisation of the perforant path input to the dentate gyrus induces a long-term potentiation (LTP) of both the population EPSP and the population spike. Plots of the EPSP-spike (E-S) relation over a number of stimulus intensities typically reveals that a shift to the left of this relation, or E-S potentiation, also occurs (Bliss & Lømo, 1973; Andersen, Sundberg, Sveen, Swann & Wigström, 1980). These findings suggest that LTP usually results in not only an enhanced excitatory synaptic drive onto granule cells but an increased ability to fire them as well.

Other studies have suggested that inhibitory interneurones can also support LTP (Buzsaki & Eidelberg, 1982; Misgeld & Klee, 1984). If true, such an outcome would be expected to modify the input-output properties of the dentate granule cells. Indeed, we have observed a lasting decrease in the slope of the E-S relation following LTP that is not easily explained by a simple model which ignores the local inhibitory circuitry (Abraham, Bliss & Goddard, 1985). Here we demonstrate decreases in granule cell input-output coupling following tetanisation and provide evidence that this may be due to LTP of the perforant path synapses onto inhibitory interneurones.

Experiments were performed in urethane anaesthetised rats using standard extracellular recordings in the dentate hilus and stimulation in the perforant path and contralateral hilus. Stimulus intensity series were computer controlled via programmable stimulators and consisted of an ascending-descending strength series of pulses to the perforant path. LTP was induced by either short high-frequency bursts of trains (400 Hz, 20 ms) or single trains of lower frequency and longer duration (250 Hz, 50-250 ms).

H.L. Haas G. Buzsàki (Eds.)
Synaptic Plasticity in the Hippocampus
© Springer-Verlag Berlin Heidelberg 1988

4

Our initial finding was that a series of 250 Hz tains of increasing duration resulted in an asynchronous development of EPSP and spike potentiation. The EPSP increased with repeated tetanisation in a relatively linear way, while the spike potentiation was retarded at the shorter train durations. This pattern of change induced by the weak trains included a decrease in the slope of the E-S curve, i.e. a decrease in the spike per unit EPSP at all points on the curve (Fig. 1). High strength trains produced the more commonly seen E-S potentiation (shift to the left), although a superimposed slope depression was still evident. E-S slope depression was not observed in 4/5 animals tested if picrotoxin (2 mg/kg i.p.) had been administered 30 min previously.

We next employed contralateral hilar tetanisation to block granule cell LTP, expecting any interneurone LTP to then be more easily expressed, in part because of the extra excitation of the interneurones that is generated by this input. In 6/10 animals, this procedure not only greatly reduced (granule cell) EPSP potentiation but also caused a reduction in spike amplitude below baseline values, even when the EPSP was slightly potentiated. This corresponded to a shift to the right of the E-S curve, with either an unchanged or decreased slope.

These data, suggestive of LTP of the perforant path-interneurone synapses, are further supported by preliminary findings from an extracellular unit study. So far four putative feed-forward inhibitory interneurones have been studied, all identified by various electrophysiological criteria including the ability to discharge with a lower threshold and shorter latency than the population spike. All four cells demonstrated a decreased threshold for discharge following perforant path tetanisation that lasted for several hours.

Whether inhibitory interneurones demonstrate LTP is an important point with respect to both the mechanism and the functional significance of this phenomenon. Hippocampal interneurones are generally regarded to be aspinous. Thus mechanistic explanations of LTP (at least for these cells) can not rely on spine shape changes as a determining factor. Perhaps more importantly, since the feed-forward inhibition engaged by afferent volleys regulates the resulting granule cell discharge, potentiation of this inhibitory pathway should decrease granule cell input-output coupling, particularly under conditions of low LTP of granule cell inputs. Our data indicate that these conditions may be met simply by the occurrence of weak trains of afferent impulses. Thus while LTP may continue to be viewed as a synaptic potentiation process, under the right conditions it may nonetheless alter the balance of excitation and inhibition such that a net depression of the population output will ensue.

Supported by the New Zealand Medical Research Council.

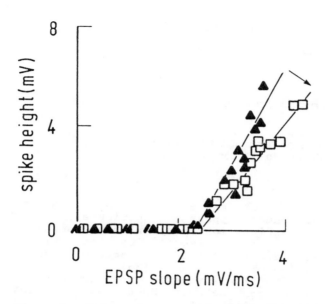

Figure 1. E-S curves made before (triangles) and 15 min after (squares) three 250 Hz trains of 170 ms. Note the potentiation of the EPSP but reduced slope of the E-S curve. (Adapted from Kairiss, Abraham, Bilkey & Goddard, 1985).

REFERENCES

Abraham, W.C., Bliss, T.V.P. & Goddard, G.V. J. Physiol. 1985, 363: 335-349.
Andersen, P., Sundberg, S.H., Sveen, O., Swann, J.W. & Wigström, H. J. Physiol. 1980, 302: 463-482.
Bliss, T.V.P. & Lømo, T. J. Physiol. 1973, 232: 331-356.
Buzsaki, G. & Eidelberg, E. J. Neurophysiol. 1982, 48: 597-607.
Kairiss, E.W., Abraham, W.C., Bilkey, D.K. & Goddard, G.V. Brain Res. 1987, 401: 87-94.
Misgeld, U. & Klee, M.R. in Sensor-motor Integration in the Nervous System, Experimental Brain Research, Supplement 9. 1984, pp. 325-332.

Frequency Potentiation and Habituation in Hippocampal Area CA1.

U. HEINEMANN, B. HAMON, R.S.G. JONES, G. KOEHR, J.D.C. LAMBERT, G. RAUSCHE, and P. SCHUBERT

Institut für normale und pathologische Physiologie, Universität Köln, Robert-Koch-Strasse 39, 5000 Köln 1, Federal Republic of Germany

Pre- and postsynaptic factors as well as changes in the extracellular microenvironment appear to contribute to frequency potentiation and habituation in synaptic transmission from Schaffer collaterals and commissural fibers onto hippocampal pyramidal cells. Presynaptic calcium accumulation as well as changes in [Ca]o, [K]o and [Mg]o could well contribute to such adaptive alterations in synaptic coupling in addition to interactions between NMDA and Non-NMDA receptors for glutamate and aspartate.

During repetitive electrical stimulation an increase in postsynaptic responses is often observed (frequency potentiation, FP). In peripheral synapses FP usually results from Ca accumulation in presynaptic endings. In central synapses pharmacological evidence points to a role of NMDA-receptors for glutamate and aspartate (1,2). FP may be present only early during a stimulus. Later it can be replaced by frequency habituation (FH), i.e. a reduction of evoked potential amplitudes. We have employed ion sensitive/reference electrodes and intracellular recording techniques to study mechanisms involved in these adaptative changes. The experiments were performed on area CA1 of rat hippocampal slices treated with different perfusion media. The experimental approach is described in detail elsewhere (3).

During repetitive electrical stimulation of the type which induces LTP, rises in [K]o to 12 mM, decreases in [Ca]o by up to 0.6 mM, in [Mg]o by up to 0.3 mM and in [Cl]o as well as [Na]o by up to 12 mM can be observed in area CA1 of rat hippocampal slices. Ionic changes show a distinct laminar profile with most ionic changes being largest in the stratum pyramidale (SP) of rat hippocampal slices. We consequently studied effects of variations in extracellular electrolytes on synaptic transmission in area CA1.

Lowering of [Ca]o lead to a reduction of both, EPSP's and IPSP's recorded intracellularly in postsynaptic elements. When Ca was very much lowered, all synaptic transmission was blocked. The Ca level at which IPSP's were blocked was higher than that of EPSP's and the balance between synaptic excitation and inhibition was varied during washout of Ca.

H.L. Haas   G. Buzsàki (Eds.)
Synaptic Plasticity in the Hippocampus
© Springer-Verlag Berlin Heidelberg 1988

Consequently, at intermediate levels of Ca orthodromic stimulation evoked epileptiform discharges. A reason for the different sensitivity of EPSP's and IPSP's to variations in [Ca]o could be found in the fact that a disynaptic pathway is more sensitive to changes in presynaptic Ca uptake than a monosynaptic pathway. In addition, lowering of [Ca]o has like lowering [Mg]o potentiating effects on NMDA-receptor mediated responses. This was investigated by studying the alterations of NMDA induced ionic signals and associated field potentials. While lowering Mg could amplify these signals by a factor of 5, lowering Ca could double NMDA signals. Quis signals were found to be little affected. Enhanced utilisation of NMDA receptors during washout of Ca would contribute to the shift in the balance between EPSP's and IPSP's in favour of excitation. Lowering of [Ca]o and [Mg]o further reduces the threshold for generation of action potentials. probably via diminished surface charge screening. Experimental test suggests this effect to be small (3.5).

Lowering [Mg]o in the presence of 1.6 mM Ca had also effects on synaptic transmission. Decreasing [Mg]o from 2 to 1 mM augmented postsynaptic responses and shifted the input/output curve to the left. This effect was not antagonized by 2-APV suggesting that it is due to enhanced presynaptic Ca-entry with subsequently enhanced transmitter release. Interestingly, NMDA-evoked postsynaptic responses where already augmented by such decreases in [Mg]o. Synaptic potentials became much enhanced by lowering Mg concentration to levels below 0.5 mM. Then EPSP's showed an enhanced NMDA-sensitive component. At levels below 0.1 mM spontaneous and evoked epileptiform activity developed which was clearly suppressed by NMDA receptor antagonists. We conclude that changes in [Mg]o are marginally involved in frequency potentiation.

Changes in [K]o also had interesting effects on synaptic transmission. The level at which synaptic transmission was blocked, was clearly dependent on the [K]o. It was 0.24 mM in the presence of 5 mM K and about 0.5 mM in the presence of 3 and 8 mM potassium. This surprising nonlinearity of block of synaptic transmission could result from depolarizing inactivation of sodium currents in presynaptic endings in high potassium medium and/or from rectifying characteristics of K channels. The well known enhancement of postsynaptic responses in high K media must therefore result from the reduction of efficacy of K outward currents, be they mediated by GABA-B-receptors or be they dependent on membrane potentials.

When Ca is lowered to levels between 0.1 and 0.2 mM, Ca concentration changes can still be observed upon activation of Schaffer collaterals and commissural fibers. These are no longer largest in SP. The maximum decrease is usually found in stratum radiatum. Various means were found to be effective in augmenting this presynaptic Ca entry. These include treatment with 4-AP and elevations in [K]o from 3 to 5 mM. Other K-channel blocking agents were less effective in augmenting presynaptic Ca entry. When Ca levels were in the range of 0.2 mM, consequent treatment with 4-AP (100 uM) could recover some synaptic transmission. When this treatment was combined with adenosine action antagonists such as theophylline and adenosinedeaminase synaptic transmission recovered even more. Interestingly, the recovery occured only late during a stimulus train suggesting that this recovery was due to presynaptic Ca accumulation. If this effect is present in low Ca medium it should be stronger in normal Ca medium and contribute significantly to frequency facilitation.

Subsequently enhanced glutamate release should then lead to enhanced EPSP's and result in partial activation of NMDA-receptors due to a removal of the voltage dependent block which Mg ions exert on NMDA operated ionophores (4). This should lead to a further enhancement of EPSP's. To test this possibility, we investigated the effect of predepolarization of nerve cells by quissqualate or kainate and found a considerable enhancement of NMDA responses and vice versa an enhancement by NMDA on quis responses. This enhancement was still present when responses were recorded in low Mg medium, containing 2-APV and ketamine suggesting the possibility of allosteric effects of NMDA on quis- and kainate receptors. Taken together, our findings indicate that presynaptic transmitter release is enhanced during repetitive stimulation. This would help to relieve the block exerted by Mg ions on NMDA-receptors near resting membrane potentials. Overspill of transmitter from the synaptic cleft would in addition activate extrasynaptic NMDA-receptors explaining the slow rise time of synaptic NMDA-components. Ca entry into postsynaptic elements mediated by NMDA-receptors and voltage dependent Ca channels may be instrumental in inducing LTP. Later habituation could result from adenosine accumulation, depressing presynaptic Ca entry. Ca dependent activation of K conductances as well as activation of an electrogenic pump may also contribute to habituation.

Supported by DFG grant He 1128/2-4.

References

1. Collingridge GL, Kehl SJ, McLennan H (1983). J Physiol. 334:19-31
2. Herron CE, Lester RA, Coan EJ, Collingridge GL (1986). Nature 322:265-268
3. Mody I, Lambert JDC and Heinemann U (1987). J. Neurophys. 57:869-888.
4. Nowak L, Bregestovski P, Ascher P, Herbert A, Prochiantz A, (1984). Nature 307:462-465
5. Yaari Y, Konnerth A, Heinemann U (1986). J Neurophysiol 56:424-436

Changes in Synaptic Transmission Evoked in the "In Vitro" Hippocampal Slice by a Brief Decrease of $[Mg^{++}]_o$: A Correlate for Long-Term Potentiation?

M. Avoli, C. Drapeau, and G. Kostopoulos

Montreal Neurological Institute and Department of Neurology and Neurosurgery, McGill University, 3801 University Street, Montréal, Québec, H3A 2B4, Canada

Perfusion of hippocampal slices with Mg^{++} free Ringer for 20-30 min evoked an increased responsiveness of CA1 pyramidal cells to stratum radiatum stimulation up to 3 hours after reintroduction of the control Ringer. This potentiation was not observed when the NMDA antagonist APV (50-100uM) was present in the Mg^{++} free Ringer. However, once the potentiation has been initiated it was no longer affected by subsequent application of similar doses of APV.

Long term potentiation (LTP), a mechanism possibly underlying learning and memory, is a phenomenon in which tetanic stimulation of a set of input fibers potentiates synaptic transmission in that pathway for several hours or days [1,3]. The initiation of LTP in the hippocampus depends upon the activation of N-methyl-D-aspartate (NMDA) receptors [2,7,9], a specific class of receptors for the excitatory aminoacid glutamate exhibiting a peculiar dependency on membrane potential in becoming active only at depolarized levels. This property is related to the presence of Mg^{++} in the extracellular space [8]. Thus the EPSP generated by CA1 pyramidal cells in response to stratum (s.) radiatum stimulation increases in amplitude and is prolonged upon perfusion with Mg^{++} free Ringer [5,6]. The present experiments were aimed at further characterizing the changes in excitatory synaptic transmission occurring in the CA1 subfield when the $[Mg^{++}]_o$ is brought to near zero value.

Experiments were performed on hippocampal slices (450um thick) from brains of adult, male, Sprague-Dawley rats (150-300g). The composition of the Ringer was (mM): NaCl 124, KCl 2, KH_2PO_4 1.25, $MgSO_4$ 2 or 0, $CaCl_2$ 2 or 4, $NaHCO_3$ 26 and glucose 10. Glass micropipettes filled with 4M NaCl were used for extracellular recordings in the s. radiatum and s. pyramidale of the CA1 subfield. Constant current anodal stimuli were delivered at 0.2-0.05Hz through sharpened and insulated tungsten electrodes placed in the s. radiatum to activate the Schaffer collateral, commissural pathway. DL-2-amino-5-phosphonovalerate (APV,50-100uM) (Sigma) was applied in the bath.

Perfusion of the slices with Mg^{++} - free Ringer for 20-30 min evoked in 19 experiments a potentiation of the responses of hippocampal pyramidal cells to stimulation of the Schaffer collateral, commissural pathway. As shown in figure 1A, the extracellular EPSP recorded in the apical dendrites displayed a shorter rising time, an increase in amplitude and a prolonged decay. These changes were characterized at the soma by the appearance of a population spike in response to orthodromic stimuli which were below

H.L. Haas G. Buzsàki (Eds.)
Synaptic Plasticity in the Hippocampus
© Springer-Verlag Berlin Heidelberg 1988

threshold in the control Ringer while at higher intensity of stimulation the population spike increased in amplitude and/or was followed by the appearance of a second one.

The excitability increase evoked by the application of Mg^{++} free Ringer could only be in part reversed by perfusing the hippocampal slice with control Ringer. This LTP of synaptic transmission in the CA1 subfield was observed up to 185min after reintroduction of control Ringer and was clearer for stimuli in a range of intensity which was below threshold for generating a population spike before perfusion with Mg^{++} free Ringer (Fig.1).

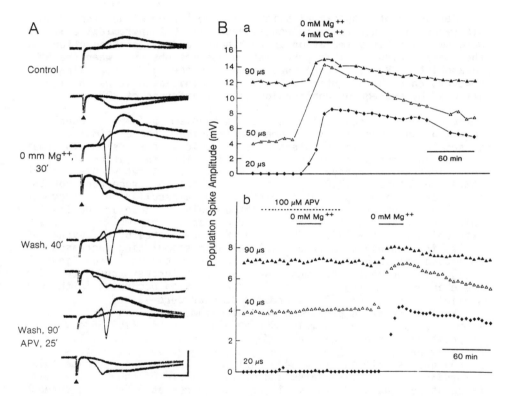

Fig.1: A: Responses of CA1 hippocampal pyramidal cells to stmulation of s. radiatum (▲). Two different intensities of stimulation (20 and 60us) are shown. In each sample the upper trace is recorded in s. pyramidale, the lower trace in s. radiatum. Calibrations: 4ms,4mV. **B: a:** Amplitudes of the population spikes evoked by s. radiatum stimulation before, during and after a transient perfusion of the hippocampal slice with Mg++ free Ringer containing 4mM Ca++. **b:** Amplitudes of the population spikes evoked by s. radiatum stimulation in four different types of Ringer as shown in the upper part of the diagram. In both **a** and **b** three different intensities of stimulations were used.

Furthermore the above described changes were also observed when the concentration of Ca^{++} in the Mg^{++} free Ringer was increased to 4mM to compensate for the decrease in divalent cations concentration (Fig.1B, upper panel). However, the changes evoked by Mg^{++} free Ringer were observed in only 8 of 13 experiments where APV was perfused with Mg^{++} free Ringer. Furthermore the increase in responsiveness observed in these 8 cases disappeared upon reintroduction of control Ringer (Fig.1B, lower panel).

In the light of these findings it appeared of interest to assess whether the maintenance of the LTP induced by Mg^{++} free Ringer could be related to the disclosure of NMDA receptors which were non operant in control conditions. In 6 experiments APV did not affect the amplitude of the population spikes evoked by orthodromic stimuli either in control or in the potentiated state while being capable of blocking the induction of the Mg^{++} - free induced LTP.

These experiments demonstrate that LTP can be evoked in the CA1 subfield by a brief perfusion of the slices with Mg^{++} free Ringer. Furthermore, the LTP does not occur in the presence of APV suggesting that the initiation of this phenomenon depends upon the activation of NMDA receptors resulting from the removal of Mg^{++} from the extracellular space. Finally our data indicate that NMDA receptors are not responsible for the maintenance of the increase in synaptic responsiveness since APV appears to have no effect on a pre-existing potentiation. The possibility that the reported phenomenon is caused by a slow reequilibration of the Mg^{++} in the extracellular space following reintroduction of control Ringer appears improbable. The time required to observe the changes evoked by the Mg^{++} free Ringer in the present experiments was usually shorter than 15min and one would expect the replacing process to be even faster since the antagonist effect of Mg^{++} on the NMDA receptors is detected at concentration of 1mM [5].

The role played by NMDA receptors in the initiation of LTP evoked by tetanic stimulation in the hippocampus rests on the demonstration that this phenomenon does not occur in the presence of the specific antagonist APV [2,7,9]. Furthermore it has been recently shown that the increased release of endogenous glutamate associated with LTP evoked by tetanic stimulation in the dentate gyrus is blocked by APV [4]. The present experiments further demonstrate the involvement of NMDA receptors in the induction of LTP. At the same time they also show that the maintenance of LTP is not caused by NMDA activated conductances.

Acknowledgement: This work was supported by the Medical Research Council of Canada (MRC Grant MA-8109 to Dr. M. Avoli).

References

1. Bliss TVP ad Lomo T, J Physiol (Lond), 232 (1973) 331-356.
2.   Collingridge GL, Kehl SJ and McLennan H, J Physiol (Lond) 334 (1983) 33-46.
3. Douglas RM and Goddard GV, Brain Res 86 (1975) 205-215.
4. Errington ML, Lynch MA and Bliss TVP, Neuroscience 20 (1987) 279-284.
5. Herron CE, Lester RAJ, Coan EJ and Collingridge GL, Neurosci Lett 60 (1985) 19-23.
6. Herron CE, Lester RAJ, Coan EJ and Collingridge GL, Nature (Lond) 322 (1986) 265-268.
7. Morris RGM, Anderson E, Lynch GS and Baudry M, Nature (Lond) 219 (1986) 774-776.
8. Novak L, Bregostovski P, Ascher P, Herbet A and Prochiantz A, Nature (Lond) 307 (1984) 462-465.
9. Wingström H, Gustafsson B and Huang YY, Neuroscience 17 (1986) 1105-1115.

Postsynaptic Mechanisms in the Potentiation of Synaptic Responses

K. L. Zbicz and F. F. Weight

Section of Electrophysiology, LPPS, National Institute on Alcohol Abuse and Alcoholism, Rockville, MD 20852, USA

ABSTRACT

The membrane mechanisms underlying the postsynaptic potentiation of synaptic responses by muscarinic receptor activation were investigated in CA3 pyramidal neurons of hippocampus using single-electrode voltage-clamp. The application of muscarine inhibited both inward Ca^{2+} current and a slowly developing, persistent Ca^{2+}-dependent outward current.

INTRODUCTION

Long-lasting potentiation of synaptic transmission by postsynaptic mechanisms has previously been described[12]. Fast EPSPs are increased in both amplitude and duration during the muscarinic postsynaptic action of the neurotransmitter acetylcholine in sympathetic neurons. A similar potentiation of fast EPSPs is observed during a long-lasting peptide-mediated postsynaptic response. The enhancement of fast EPSP amplitude increases the probability of postsynaptic action potential generation, and thus increases the efficacy of impulse transmission at the synapses. The primary membrane mechanism underlying this long-lasting potentiation of synaptic transmission is a decrease in membrane K^+ conductance[14]. Brown & Adams[3] have proposed that the K^+ current that is decreased by muscarinic action is a voltage-dependent K^+ current, termed M-current. Halliwell & Adams[8] have also attributed muscarinic action in hippocampal pyramidal neurons to the suppression of M-current. However, Bernardo & Prince[1], and Cole & Nicoll[6] have suggested that the effects of muscarinic agonists involve Ca^{2+}-dependent K^+ conductances. We have investigated the K^+ current that is suppressed by muscarinic agonists in CA3 hippocampal pyramidal neurons using single-electrode voltage clamp. Our studies indicate that a slowly activating, persistent Ca^{2+}-dependent outward current is inhibited by muscarinic activation.

METHODS AND RESULTS

Slices of guinea pig hippocampus (400–450μ) were held submerged in a transverse flow tissue chamber at 31°C, as described previously[15]. Cells in the CA3 stratum pyramidale were impaled with a single microelectrode (10–25 Mohms) filled with either 3M CsCl or 3M KCl solutions. Depolarizing steps to potentials positive to −40 mV produced a gradually increasing outward current in neurons impaled with either type of microelectrode. However, the slowly increasing outward current was

H.L. Haas   G. Buzsàki (Eds.)
Synaptic Plasticity in the Hippocampus
© Springer-Verlag Berlin Heidelberg 1988

much more distinct in CsCl filled cells due, most likely, to suppression of other outward currents. Most of the experiments in this study were performed using CsCl filled microelectrodes. Tetrodotoxin ($2x10^{-7}$–$2x10^{-6}$ M) was present in the bathing solution in all experiments.

After impalement with a CsCl-filled microelectrode, a reduction in depolarization activated outward current developed over a period of 10–15 min. The outward current which remained in Cs^+-loaded neurons appeared to activate between –40 and –30 mV, and gradually increased over a period of 0.5 to 1.5 sec. Upon repolarization, an outward tail current was observed which decayed with a single time-constant of between 200 and 400 msec. The outward current and associated tail current appeared to be Ca^{2+}-dependent, as they were greatly reduced or abolished by application of the divalent Ca^{2+}-channel blockers Co^{2+} and Mn^{2+}, and by the application of Ca^{2+}-free solutions. There was no evidence of a significant contribution to the recorded current by other outward currents after Cs^+-loading. The Ca^{2+}-dependent outward current was also greatly reduced by application of 10 mM TEA, but not by 0.5 mM 4–AP. This current resembles the Ca^{2+}-activated K^+ current described in these cells by Brown & Griffith[4]. The slow outward current and tail current were also greatly reduced or blocked by the application of Ba^{2+} (0.2–2 mM).

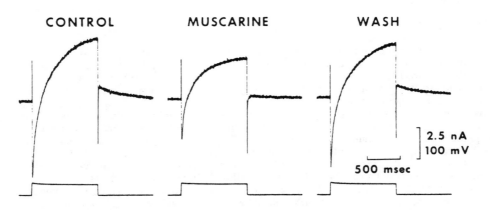

FIG. 1. Effect of muscarine on currents in a CA3 pyramidal neuron.

Figure 1 illustrates the effect of 20 uM muscarine on the currents activated in a Cs^+-loaded neuron stepped from –40 mV to –15 mV. As was typical for these neurons, depolarization activated a large inward current followed by a slowly developing, persistent large outward current. A slowly decaying outward tail current was observed upon repolarization. The application of muscarine reduced the initial inward Ca^{2+} current, as well as both the outward current and the tail current. These effects were reversed by washing in the normal bathing solution for 15 min. However, when neurons were bathed in a Ca^{2+}-free solution containing 3 mM Co^{2+} or 4 mM Mn^{2+}, the application of muscarine did not produce a depression of the remaining outward current. In neurons impaled with microelectrodes containing KCl, muscarine produced an outward shift in the initial depolarization activated current and a suppression of the slowly increasing, persistent outward current and associated tail current.

DISCUSSION

Hippocampal pyramidal neurons generate several membrane currents which appear to play important roles in regulating the response of the neurons to external stimuli. The activation of these currents usually begins at membrane potentials negative to spike threshold, and the currents have relatively long duration effects on membrane conductance and potential, when compared to the currents involved in spike generation. In pyramidal neurons of hippocampus, several currents have been described which, by means of pharmacological manipulation, have been shown to profoundly affect the excitability of these neurons. Among the first 'modulatory' currents described were the inward Ca^{2+} and outward Ca^{2+}-activated K^+ currents in invertebrate neurons. These currents were suggested to be the basis for intrinsic spiking patterns, such as bursting, and patterns in response to external stimuli, such as accomodation. Currents analogous to these have since been demonstrated in hippocampal pyramidal neurons[4,5]. Subsequent observations indicate that neurotransmitters can modify various currents in CNS neurons[1,2,3 6,9,11].

A long-lasting potentiation of synaptic transmission is associated with inhibition of membrane K^+ current by muscarinic receptor activation in sympathetic neurons[12,14]. Brown & Adams[3] proposed that the K^+ current that is reduced by muscarinic activation is a voltage-activated K^+ current they called M-current. In hippocampal pyramidal neurons, Halliwell & Adams[8] reported that muscarinic activation depressed outward current activated by depolarization and attributed this effect to suppression of M-current. On the other hand, on the basis of current-clamp experiments, Bernardo & Prince[1], and Cole & Nicoll[6] have suggested that muscarinic actions may involve Ca^{2+}-dependent K^+ conductances. Our results suggest that the effects of muscarinic agonists on outward current can be expained, at least in part, by effects on Ca^{2+}-dependent outward current. Similar effects of muscarinic agonists have been observed in other neuron types[9,13]. Our observation that Ba^{2+} inhibits the Ca^{2+}-dependent outward current suggests that the effects of Ba^{2+} that were attributed to suppression of M-current[8], can also be explained by effects on Ca^{2+}-dependent outward current.

While the ion species carrying the charge for the slow outward current in Cs^+-loaded neurons has not been established, it is likely that it is mediated by the slow Ca^{2+}-activated K^+ conductance described by Brown & Griffith[4], due to the similarities in time course and pharmacological sensitivity. It should also be noted that the reduction of inward Ca^{2+} current by muscarine suggests that the decrease in Ca^{2+}-dependent outward current that results from muscarinic receptor activation may be due to inhibition of Ca^{2+} current.

REFERENCES

1. Bernardo, L.S. & Prince, D.A. J. Neuroscience 2: 415-423, 1982.
2. Bernardo, L.S. & Prince, D.A. Brain Res. 249: 333-344, 1982.
3. Brown, D.A. & Adams, P.R. Nature 283: 673-676, 1980.
4. Brown, D.A. & Griffith, W.H. J. Physiol. 337: 287-301, 1983.
5. Brown, D.A. & Griffith, W.H. J. Physiol. 337: 303-320, 1983.
6. Cole, A.E. & Nicoll, R.A. J. Physiol. 352: 173-188, 1984.
7. Grafe, P., Mayer, C.J. & Wood, J.D. J. Physiol. 305: 235-248, 1980.
8. Halliwell, J.V. & Adams, P.R. Brain Res. 250: 71-92, 1982.
9. North, R.A. & Tokimasa, T. J. Physiol. 342: 253-266, 1983.

10. Pellmar, T.C.   J. Neurophysiol. 55: 727-738, 1986.
11. Sah, P., French, C.R. & Gage, P. Neurosci. Lett. 60: 295-300, 1985.
12. Schulman, J.A. & Weight, F.F.   Science 194: 1437-1439, 1976.
13. Tokimasa, T.   Brain Res. 344: 134-141, 1985.
14. Weight, F.F. & Votava, J.   Science 170: 755-757, 1970.
15. Zbicz, K.L. & Weight, F.F.   J. Neurophysiol. 53: 1038-1058, 1985.

* Current address: Armed Forces Radiobiological Research Institute,
                     National Naval Medical Center, Bethesda, MD 20814.

Postsynaptic Mechanisms May Regulate Synaptic Strength by Controlling Synapse Lifetimes

R. MALINOW and H. T. CLINE

Departments of Physiology and Biology, Yale University, New Haven, CT 06513, USA

Results are presented showing that postsynaptic hyperpolarization of CA1 neurons during tetanization reversibly blocks induction of long-term potentiation (LTP). Others have shown that pharmacologic blockade of N-methyl-D-aspartate (NMDA) receptors blocks LTP and that the NMDA receptor requires both membrane depolarization and agonist to be activated. Together these results imply that postsynaptic NMDA receptor activation is necessary to trigger LTP. Does NMDA activation affect the strength of existing synapses or is an anatomical redistribution of synapses effected? Data from a different system (frog retinotectal projection) suggests that NMDA activation is critical to selective synapse maintenance. One may speculate that similar mechanisms operate in the hippocampus.

Until recently, no direct evidence supported the hypothesis that postsynaptic membrane potential controlled the development of LTP. We se out to determine if postsynaptic hyperpolarization during the tetanizing conditioning stimulus (TCS) could block LTP. The main problem was to control the synaptic membrane potential in the dendrites while recording from the cell body. Thus we attempted to a) minimize the distance between the synapses activated and the cell body; b) maximize the hyperpolarizing current passage during the TCS without damaging the cell; and c) minimize the strength of the TCS while still inducing LTP. To satisfy there a) afferents were stimulated which, based on the generally laminar arrangement of afferents, were predicted to run close to the cell body; b) 3 nA of hyperpolarizing current was passed in (test) cells during the TCS and cells were monitored with respect to membrane potential, chance in input resistance and subsequent ability to undergo LTP; d) a relatively low frequency stimulation was used (30 Hz X 5sec) and simultaneous intracellular recording from a neighboring (control) cell showed that the TCS was indeed sufficient to induce LTP.

The results, shown in Figures 1 and 2, reveal that the epsp's of the (test) cells which had been hyperpolarized during the TCS showed no significant increase in amplitude. A nearby (control) cell did undergo LTP demonstrating that the TCS was sufficient. When those test cells (or cells which had been hyperpolarized by the passage of 3 nA of current) were subsequently delivered a TCS in the absence of hyperpolarizing current, LTP ensued. The ability to undergo LTP and the absence of a change in input resistance (< 5%) demonstrates the continued health of test cells following a transient 3 nA hyperpolarizing current passage.

These results indicated that postsynaptic depolarization during the TCS is necessary for the induction of LTP. Others have shown that blockade of the NMDA subclass of glutamate receptor prevents LTP (1). However, such pharmacological experiments cannot localize the site of block: pre- or postsynaptic. Since the NMDA receptor requires membrane depolarization and agonist binding to be activated, our results imply that postsynaptic NMDA receptor activation is necessary to trigger LTP.

H. L. Haas   G. Buzsàki (Eds.)
Synaptic Plasticity in the Hippocampus
© Springer-Verlag Berlin Heidelberg 1988

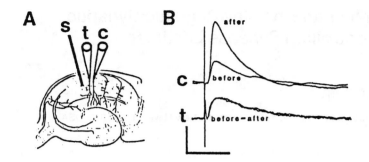

Fig 1 A. Diagram of a hippocampal slice showing the location of the bipolar extracellular stimulating electrode (s), the intracellular electrode in the control cell
(c), and the intracellular electrode in the test cell (t). B. The upper traces show
an intracellular recording from a control cell which did not receive any current
passage during the TCS.
Lower traces show a simultaneous intracellular recording from a nearby test cell
(t) which received passage of a 3-nA hyperpolarizing current during the TCS. Each
trace is the average of five successive responses 4 s apart recorded immediately
before and 10 minutes after the TCS.

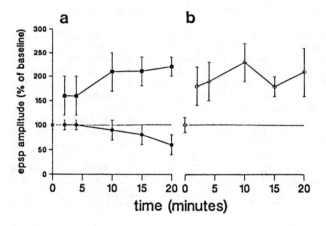

Fig 2 A. Hyperpolarization during the TCS prevents LTP. Filled squares represent
control responses from cells not hyperpolarized during the TCS. Filled circles represent simultaneous responses from test cell hyperpolarized by 3-nA during the
TCS. B. Transient hyperpolarization before TCS does not prevent LTP. Cells were
hyperpolarized by 3-nA and then delivered a TCS.

What does NMDA activation effect? The data presented here suggest that (at least part of) the trigger for LTP activation lies postsynaptically. Are pre- or postsynaptic changes responsible for the increase in synaptic strength? Others have data suggesting both pre- and postsynaptic changes following LTP (2-8). One hypothesis consistent with these data is that postsynaptic NMDA activation increases the lifetime of normally transient synapses. A different system in which anatomical changes are more easily monitored may shed light on this issue.

In surgically produced three-eyed Rana pipiens tadpoles, retinal ganglion cells (RGC) from the normal and supernumerary eyes project to the same optic tectum and their terminals segregate into stereotyped eye-specific stripes resembling the ocular dominance columns seen n higher vertebrates (9,10). These stripe configurations are maintained as the RGC afferents progress across the tectum during normal development. Therefore some mechanisms must exist for maintaining stripes (RGC terminal segregation) in the face of the continual making and breaking of synaptic connections known to occur during retino-tectal development. Investigators have suggested that neighboring afferent co-activity is crucial to eye-specific segregation and that this co-activity is sensed by a post-synaptic mechanism (11,12). We tested whether NMDA activation is necessary for the maintenance of these eye-specific stripes by chronically exposing the tecta of three-eyed tadpoles to aminophosphono-valeric acid (APV), a specific antagonist of the NMDA receptor (13). APV (1 mM, 0.1 mM or 0.01 mM) was suspended in the polymer Elvax, and slices were implanted over the optic tecta of three-eyed tadpoles. After 2.5-4 weeks, the supernumerary retinal projection was labeled with standard horseradish peroxidase techniques. In sham-operated tadpoles (Fig 3a), the supernumerary retinal afferents terminate in eye-specific interdigitating bands ~200 uM wide, oriented along the rostrocaudal axis of the tectum. In contrast, the supernumerary retina of animals treated with APV for 4 weeks projects evenly over the tectum (Fig 3b). Control experiments show that this effect is reversible (with removal of the APV), and is not due to a toxic effect of the drug. Preliminary data suggest that APV does not block synaptic transmission. These results suggest that activation of the NMDA receptor allows tectal neurons to recognize and maintaining coactive afferent synapses, while inappropriate inputs are lost (14).

Although the systems are markedly different, based on these results we may speculate on mechanisms operating in the hippocampus. We suggest that in the hippocampus there is normally a continual making and breaking of synapses and that one of the factors determining the lifetime of a synapse is postsynaptic activation of NMDA receptors. With tetanic stimulation, NMDA receptors are activated leading to longer lifetimes of those synapses already formed and stimulated. With the continual formation of new synapses (which may or may not be under NMDA control) and longer maintenance of older synapses, the effective synaptic strength increases.

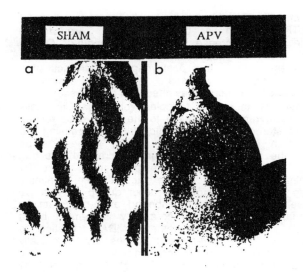

Fig 3 A. A tectum from a sham-operated animal implanted with FITC-Elvax shows the stereotypical striped pattern representing the segregation of the supernumerary retinal afferents from the afferents of the normal eye. The segregation of the inputs is not altered by the operation nor the mechanical effect of the Elvax on the tectum (n=5). B. A tectum from an animal treated with APV (10 uM) for 4 weeks displays complete overlap of the supernumerary and normal retinal projections.

References

1. Herron, CE et al (1986) Nature 322:331-356.
2. Bliss, TVP & Lomo, T (1973) J Physiol, Lond 302:463-482.
3. Dolphin, AC et al (1982) Nature 297:496-498.
4. Andersen, P et al (1980) J Physiol, Lond. 302:463-482.
5. McNaughton BL et al (1978) Brain Res 157:277-293.
6. Lynch G et al (1983) Nature 305:719-721.
7. Dunwiddie, T & Lynch, G (1978) J Physiol, Lond 276:353-367.
8. Baudry et al (1981) Science 212:937-938.
9. Constantine-Paton, M & Law M (1978) Science 202:639-641.
10. Law, M & Constantine-Paton, M (1981) J Neurosci. 1:741-759.
11. Constantine-Paton, M & Reh, T (1985) in Neurobiology: Molecular Biological Approaches to Understanding Neuronal Function and Development (ed P. O'Lague)
12. Changeuz, JP & Danchin, A (1976) Nature 264:705-712.
13. Davies, J & Watkins, J (1982) Brain Res 235:378-386.

Long-Term Potentiation of Inhibitory Responses in the Dentate Gyrus

R. J. Racine, M. deJonge, and T. Kennedy

Department of Psychology, McMaster University, Hamilton, Ontario, L8S 4K1, Canada

Repeated epileptogenic stimulation (kindling) of the perforant path or the dentate gyrus results in a long-lasting potentiation of 2 components of inhibition as measured from field responses using a double pulse technique. This potentiation of inhibitory responses does not accompany normal LTP of the excitatory input, but preliminary experiments indicate that it may be induced by non-epileptogenic stimulation applied directly to the hilar region. The mechanism underlying this effect appears to be an increase in the number of GABA and benzodiazepine receptors.

Appropriate patterns of activation can produce synaptic potentiation in excitatory projection pathways such as the perforant path between the entorhinal cortex and the dentate gyrus (Bliss and Lomo, 1973). Repeated epileptogenic stimulation (kindling) produces similar potentiation effects (Racine, et. al., 1983).

Using the field potential recording technique, it is possible to monitor inhibitory as well as excitatory events over long periods of time. If a second pulse is applied to the perforant path within 30 msec or so of the first pulse, the response triggered by the second pulse will fall within the period of recurrent inhibition generated by the first response. The result is that both the population EPSP and the population spike will be depressed when compared with the first response (Adamec, et. al., 1981). Although it is more difficult to interpret the results of field potential (vs intracellular) data, the paired pulse depression is appropriately sensitive to drugs which affect the function of GABAergic synapses. GABA agonists increase, and GABA antagonists decrease, the depression effect (Tuff, et. al., 1983). There is a second component of paired pulse depression which peaks at about 200-300 msec and may be related to various late afterhyperpolarization phenomena (Newberry and Nicoll, 1984).

We used the paired pulse technique to monitor inhibition as animals were kindled. We expected to see a disinhibition effect, but instead found a kindling-induced increase in paired pulse depresssion. Both the early and the late components of depression were affected (Tuff, et. al., 1983).

Although it was clear from the initial experiments that this was a long-lasting effect, we had no indication as to the rate of decay. More specifically, we did not know whether the early and late components of inhibition developed and decayed together or independently. In subsequent experiments we monitored the paired pulse depression _during_ kindling and for 4 weeks after the completion

H. L. Haas   G. Buzsàki (Eds.)
Synaptic Plasticity in the Hippocampus
© Springer-Verlag Berlin Heidelberg 1988

of kindling. One group of animals was kindled in the perforant path, another in the dentate gyrus and a third group served as a control. We found that the early component of inhibition began to show an increase almost immediately (after the first few epileptiform discharges had been triggered) and peaked within 10 days of stimulation. The late component of inhibition, on the other hand, showed no clear potentiation effect until after about 10 days of stimulation, and did not reach a peak until near the end of kindling. The picture was reversed for rate of decay. The late component was back to baseline levels in most animals after about 2 weeks. The early component decayed more slowly and was still potentiated after 4 weeks.

This "potentiation of inhibition" effect resembled other types of LTP. Its development was relatively rapid (at least for the early component of depression), and it decayed with a time course that was similar to that found for LTP in excitatory systems. If this was a real LTP-type effect, it would seem to be the first clear demonstration of such an effect involving local circuit neurons (although Buzsaki and Eidelberg, 1982, have provided evidence for an increase in feedforward inhibition following the induction of LTP in the perforant path). The next series of experiments addressed the question of whether the effect could be produced by non-epileptogenic stimulation.

If the potentiation of inhibition effect involved changes at the synapses between interneurons and granule cells, then it seemed unlikely that it would be induced during the normal induction of LTP in the perforant path. The granule cells do not discharge repetitively during typical, brief high frequency stimulation trains. This means that the interneurons are receiving no more than one action potential per synapse. This would not appear to be an optimal pattern for potentiation, if we can judge from the behavior of other systems. Nevertheless, we monitored the paired pulse effects before and after the induction of LTP in the perforant path and found that there was, in fact, no change in the level of paired pulse depression. We followed this up with a test of the effects of several other train patterns. Perhaps a lower frequency train (1-10 hz) that allowed the granule cells to follow the pulse frequency would produce a sufficient level of activation to induce potentiation in the interneurons. Again, stimulation trains applied to the perforant path were ineffective in producing changes in paired pulse depression.

Our final attempts to induce potentiation at the level of the interneurons involved direct stimulation via electrodes implanted in the region where the cell bodies are located. We reasoned that direct stimulation of the interneurons might successfully provide the pattern of activation that is necessary for the induction of synaptic potentiation. Our first experiments failed because it was almost impossible to avoid the triggering of epileptiform discharge with anything but the lowest intensity trains. We solved this problem by anesthetizing the animals before applying the stimulation trains. The paired pulse responses were monitored in the waking state before and after the application of the stimuation trains. This time, we found evidence for an increase in paired pulse depression with non-epileptogenic stimulation. We are currently attempting to replicate these results and provide an anesthetised-only control group (Kennedy, Racine, deJonge and Gilbert, in progress).

The replication of this result would provide additional evidence for plasticity at the interneuron level. The question will still remain as to whether it is the temporal pattern of activation that is critical for the potentiation of inhibition, or if the direct hilar stimulation allowed the activation of an appropriate spatial pattern of inputs (e.g. the activation of necessary modulatory inputs). If it is the temporal pattern that is critical, then under what conditions would such temporal patterns be activated?

The mechanism underlying this potentiation of inhibition effect may be postsynaptic. We measured GABA and flunitrazepam (a benzodiazepine) binding in our initial experiments (Tuff, et. al., 1983) and found evidence for an increase in the number of benzodiazepine (and possibly GABA) receptors. These results have been replicated several times. In order to confirm the viability of an LTP mechanism, however, it is necessary to demonstrate that it follows a similar time-course. In a preliminary kindling experiment we have found that GABA and benzodiazepine binding decays at about the same rate as the increased paired pulse depression (deJonge, Racine and Burnham, in progress).

REFERENCES

Adamec, R., McNaughton, B., Racine, R., and Livingston, K. Effect of diazepam (Valium) on hippocampal excitability in the cat: Action in the dentate area, Epilepsia, 1981, 22, 205-215.

Bliss, T.B.P. and Lomo, T. Long-lasting potentiation of synaptic transmission in the dentate gyrus of the anaesthetized rabbit following stimulation of the perforant path, J. Physiol. 1973, 232, 331-356.

Buzsaki, G. and Eidelberg, E. Direct afferent excitation and long-term potentiation of hippocampal interneurons, J. Neurophysiol. 1982, 49, 597-607.

deJonge, M. and Racine, R. The development and decay of kindling-induced increases in paired-pulse depression in the dentate gyrus, Brain Res. 1987 (in press).

Newberry, N. and Nicoll, R. A bicuculline-resistant inhibitory post-synaptic potential in rat hippocampal pyramidal cells in vitro, J. Physiol. 1984, 348, 239-254.

Racine, R., Milgram, N. and Hafner, S. Long-term potentiation phenomena in the rat limbic forebrain, Brain Res. 1983, 260, 217-231.

Tuff, L., Racine, R. and Adamec, R. The effects of kindling on GABA-mediated inhibition in the dentate gyrus of the rat. I. Paired-pulse depression, Brain Res. 1983, 277, 79-90.

Quantal Analysis of Synaptic Plasticity in the Hippocampus

C. YAMAMOTO, M. HIGASHIMA, and S. SAWADA

Department of Physiology, Faculty of Medicine, Kanazawa University, Kanazawa 920, Japan

Quantal analysis of synaptic transmission between mossy fibers and CA3 neurons revealed that potentiation by phorbol esters is accompanied by increases in quantal content. This indicates that phorbol esters facilitate release of neurotransmitter and thereby potentiate synaptic transmission.

In order to determine the primary site of changes underlying long-term potentiation (LTP), we developed a technique to apply quantal analysis to synapses in the hippocampus. In the present study, we analyzed, with this

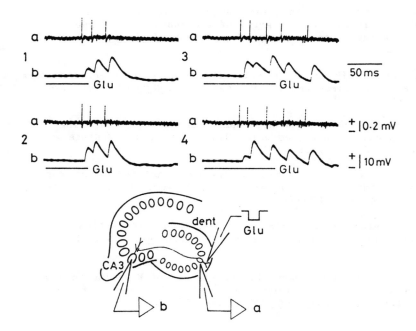

Fig. 1. Simultaneous recordings of granule cell spikes and EPSPs. Traces a show granule cell discharges and traces b EPSP trains.

H.L. Haas   G. Buzsàki (Eds.)
Synaptic Plasticity in the Hippocampus
© Springer-Verlag Berlin Heidelberg 1988

technique, a long-lasting potentiation induced by phorbol esters. Phorbol esters cause activation of protein kinase C which has been inferred to trigger the LTP (1,2).

Transvers sections (about 0.4 mm thick) of the hippocampus were prepared from the guinea pig (3). Intracellular potentials were recorded from CA3 neurons with glass microelectrodes filled with 4 M potassium acetate. Upon impalement of a CA3 neuron, a micropipette filled with 0.2 M L-glutamate (Glu) was repeatedly inserted into the granular layer to search for a spot where ejection of Glu induced a train of large excitatory postsynaptic potentials (EPSPs) in the impaled neuron at the lowest intensity (Fig. 1b). In some experiments, it was possible to record simultaneously spikes of granule cells which occurred in an one-to-one manner just before

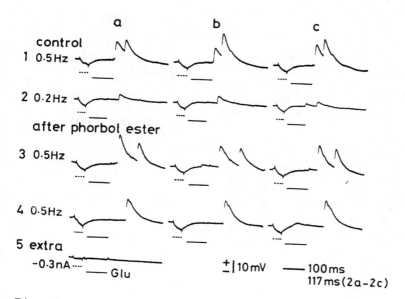

Fig. 2. EPSP trains before and during administration of PD at 0.1 μM.

individual EPSPs (Fig. 1a). This indicates that a granule cell making synaptic contacts with the impaled neuron was activated by Glu pulses and the activated granule cell induced EPSP trains in the impaled neuron.

Although simultaneous recordings of presynaptic and postsynaptic events provide convincing data, this was only rarely possible. Therefore, we recorded EPSPs for quantal analysis without presynaptic spikes. Since the failure of quantal release could no be detected in the lack of presynaptic spike recording, we took a precaution to collect the data under the condition where the transmission failure was absent. For this purpose, we selected neurons which generated large EPSPs and in which, because of frequency potentiation, the minimal amplitude of the first EPSPs in trains elicited at 0.5 or 1 nz was at least twice as large as that elicited at 0.2 Hz (Fig. 2). The first EPSPs in trains elicited at 0.5 or 1 Hz were used for quantal analysis. We think the possibility of transmission failure in these EPSPs was negligible. The rationale is as follows. Since the minimal EPSP amplitude at 0.5 or 1 Hz was more than two-times larger than that at 0.2 Hz, and since at least one quantum was released to produce a minimal EPSP at 0.2 Hz, the quantal contents were two or more throughout all trains at 0.5 or 1 Hz. EPSPs induced by a single quantum were not observed. Assuming that the distribution of the EPSP amplitude fits Poisson distribution, we may assume that the possibility of transmission failure was practically zero.

The amplitude of EPSPs fluctuated from train to train (Fig. 2). It increased gradually during administration of phorbol diacetate (PD) over a time-course of about 20 min (Fig. 2, rocords 3 and 4). More than 100 EPSP trains were recorded under each condition, the amplitudes of the first EPSPs in trains were measured and corrected for non-linear summation. The mean quantal amplitude (q) and the mean quantal content (m) were calculated from the mean and variance of the EPSP amplitude (4). In 7 neurons from which data were recorded successfully, the values of q and m were 1.1 mV and 9.7, respectively, on the average. In all of the neurons, the mean EPSP amplitudes increased under the action of PD at concentratins between 0.1 and 0.45 μM. In all of them, the values of m increased 1.5-4.3 times whereas the values of q remained unchanged or markedly decreased.

The above findings indicate that PD potentiates synaptic transmission by facilitating release of neurotransmitter.

References

1. Akers, R.F., Lovinger, D.M., Colley, P.A., Linden, D.J. and Routtenberg, A., Science, 231: 587-589, 1986.
2. Malenka, R.C., Madison, D.V. and Nicoll, R.A., Nature (London), 321: 175-177, 1986.
3. Yamamoto, C., Exp. Brain Res., 14: 423-435, 1972.
4. Yamamoto, C., Exp. Brain Res., 46: 170-176, 1982.

Quantal Analysis of Long-Term Potentiation

L. L. VORONIN

Brain Institute, Mental Health Center, Academy of Medical Sciences, 107120 Moscow, USSR

Summary: Quantal analysis was performed on evoked EPSPs recorded from hippocampal neurones in *in vivo* (rabbit) and in *in vitro* (guinea pig) preparations. In one series of experiments double pulse stimulation was used. In two other series, test stimuli with low repetition rate were given at least for 15 min before and up to 60 min after short tetanic trains which induced LTP. Two basic methods were used to calculate quantal parameters. The results of both methods point to a mainly presynaptic location of mechanisms which underly LTP and double pulse facilitation and a small (if any) participation of postsynaptic mechanisms.

Long-term potentiation (LTP) is an interesting phenomenon of hippocampal plasticity [2]. Several properties of LTP have been revealed (see [10] for review) which are similar to properties of memory and behavioural conditioning. This similarities suggest common underlying mechanisms and justify the study of LTP as an experimental model for memory. Quantitative methods based on the quantum hypothesis (see for review [7,9]) enable one to calculate parameters which can be used to characterize a synaptic connection under study: mean quantal content (m), quantal size (v) and binomial parameters (p and n). The important question of the location of LTP mechanisms could be answered by estimating if m or v changes with LTP. The aim of this presentation is to summarize our studies on quantal analysis in *in vivo* [8-11] and *in vitro* preparations [12].

Three series of experiments (A, B and C) will be reported. Series A was done on unanaesthetized rabbits according to methods previousely described [8,9]. A movable stimulating microelectrode was inserted between a recording glass microelectrode in CA3-CA4 area and a stimulating dentate gyrus macroelectrode. "Minimal" excitatory postsynaptic potentials (EPSPs) with mean amplitude (E) below 1 mV and with failures were evoked by stimulation through the microelectrode. Tetanic stimulation (a train of 5–20 s at 20 Hz) was delivered through the macroelectrode. Series B and C were done on hippocampal slices prepared from guinea pigs [5]. Aggregate EPSPs with $E > 1$ mV and minimal EPSPs were recorded in series B and C, respectively. "Quasi-stationary" plateau regions

H.L. Haas   G. Buzsàki (Eds.)
Synaptic Plasticity in the Hippocampus
© Springer-Verlag Berlin Heidelberg 1988

(see [7,9]) were determined from plots of means of 10 or 20 consecutive response amplitudes. Two basic methods (see [7–11] for details) were used to calculate quantal parameters for control (I) and post-tetanic (II and III) regions. Method 1 is based on the estimation of v_1 as the mean separation between extremal points of the amplitude histogram. The histogram was divided into classes and parameters m_1, p_1, n_1 were calculated according to established equations. According to Method 2, p_2 was obtained as a ratio of E to the maximum amplitude; m_2 was calculated from the number of failures (N_0) and the coefficient of variation; v_2 and n_2 were estimated from equations: $E = mv$ and $m = np$.

In series A, double pulse stimulation was used. In 4 of 5 neurones with significant LTP, only the second testing pulse evoked EPSP. Altogether areas of six EPSPs were measured for control (I), 2 to 5 min (II) and 6 to 12 min (III) after tetanization. The areas were then recalculated into amplitudes. The amplitude histograms shifted to the right along the abscissa after tetanization without significant changes in distances between main peaks, indicating changes in m with constant v (Fig.1A,m_1, v_1). Parameters m_2, v_2 were calculated in this series by the method of failures at $N_0 > 4$ and by the variance method if $N <= 4$. The results of Method 2 (Fig.1A,m_2, v_2) were similar to those of Method 1. Binomial parameters either increased after tetanization or distributions with uncertain n and p transformed into distributions close to binomial. Relative post-tetanic bi-

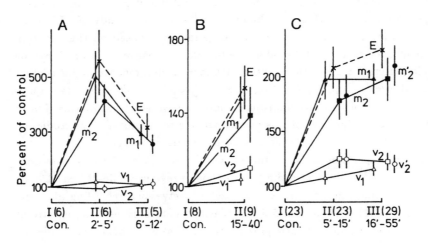

Fig.1 Changes in E, m, and v in *in vivo* (A) and *in vitro* (B,C) experiments with recording of minimal (A,C) and aggregate EPSPs (B). Post-tetanic values (II, III) were normalized to the control (I) and plotted as a percentage of the latter$\pm SEM$. Values in parenthesis are the number of measurements. See text for other notations.

nomial parameters (mean$\pm SEM, N = 8$) calculated by Method 2 as ratios to the corresponding pretetanic values were $p_2 = 1.89 \pm 0.39$ and $n_2 = 1.75 \pm 0.44$.

Because of technical reasons, it was impossible to keep neurones in stable conditions for a post-tetanic period of longer than 15 min. Hippocampal slice preparations provide a better possibility for stable recordings [4]. In a collaborative study with Kuhnt and Hess [12], we compared control quantal parameters with those recorded for a longer post-tetanic period (usually 15–30 min). Mean LTP magnitude for aggregate EPSPs recorded in 7 neurones (8 pathways, 9 post-tetanic regions) was smaller in this series (Fig.1B,E) in comparison with series A (Fig.1A) but the character of changes in m and v (Fig.1B) were basically the same. Only an insignificant trend for v to increase was found (Fig.1B,v_2). Parameter p did not change, the mean relative values being $p_1 = 0.99 \pm 0.06$ and $p_2 = 1.07 \pm 0.04$. Changes in n more closely paralleled the increase in E and m: $n_1 = 1.56 \pm 0.17$, $n_2 = 1.31 \pm 0.14$.

Series A and B indicate that the basic mechanism of both *in vivo* and *in vitro* LTP consists in an increase in m. However, a trend for v to change was seen in series B and p was not changed in this series. For more precise analysis, minimal EPSPs of 9 neurones (11 pathways, 43 post-tetanic regions) were recorded in *in vitro* preparation, mainly with double pulse stimulation. The method of failures was used for regions with $N_0 > 1\%$ of all responses and "mixed" parameters were calculated on the basis of failure and variance methods (Fig.1C,m_2', v_2'). Two post-tetanic regions (5–15 and > 15 min, up to 55 min) were analyzed. Again, mainly m changed during LTP. A small increase in v (from 7 to 20 percent, according to various methods) was also found (Fig.1C). It was statistically significant for v_1, region III ($P < 0.05$, the sign test), for v_2, region II ($P < 0.05$) and III ($P < 0.005$), for pooled data of regions II and III for the histogram and failure methods ($P < 0.05$) and not significant for all other cases. Both p and n usually increased, relative post-tetanic values for Method 2 being $p_2 = 1.32 \pm 0.05$, $n_2 = 1.40 \pm 0.06$ (N=43).

The difference in n changes for minimal and aggregate EPSPs could be understood on the basis of a relatively large number of "ineffective" connections (release sites) with very low pretetanic p values [9,10]. It could be suggested that a strong stimulus which evokes aggregate EPSPs activates a significant number of connections with a high p, so that a post-tetanic increase in p in previously ineffective connections does not influence strongly the mean p. In contrast, with excitation of a few fibres (minimal EPSPs), mainly connections with a small initial p are activated, and post-tetanic increase should be more clear.

In summary, a significant increase in m with only a small increase in v was found. Within the framework of the quantal hypothesis, our data strongly suggest a presynaptic location for LTP mechanisms, with only a small (if any) contribution of postsynaptic mechanisms. It has previously been noted [9–11] that changes m in a situation with initially ineffective synapses must be interpreted with caution [9–11]. It has been noted that ineffective synapses which make no essential contribution to the pretetanic EPSPs could increase their efficacy due to either presynaptic or subsynaptic reorganization (formation of new receptors). If this is true, our data show that the mean efficacy of one transmitter quanta for presumed "new" synapses must be about the same as that for initially effective synapses and that sensitivity of existing subsynaptic receptors (and other postsynaptic characteristics) does not change significantly during LTP. The traditional explanation of our data, based on purely presynaptic mechanisms which increase the number of quanta released per presynaptic spike, is supported by transmitter release [3,6] as well as by Ca^{2+}-uptake studies [1] and seems to be most attractive.

References: 1.Agoston DV, Kuhnt U (1986) Exp Brain Res 62:663-668. 2.Bliss TVP, Lomo T (1973) J Physiol(Lond) 232:331-356. 3.Dolphin AC, Errington ML, Bliss TVP (1983) Nature 297:496-498. 4.Kuhnt U (1984) Neurosci Lett Suppl 18:S27. 5.Kuhnt U, Kelly MJ, Schaumberg R (1979) Exp Brain Res 35:372-385. 6.Skrede KK, Malthe-Sorenssen D (1981) Brain Res 208:436-441. 7.Voronin LL (1979) Neurophysiology(Kiev) 11:491-505. 8.Voronin LL (1981) Adv Physiol Sci 36:165-174. 9.Voronin L.L. (1982) Analysis of Plastic Properties of the Central Nervous System (in Russian), Metsniereba, Tbilisi. 10.Voronin LL (1983) Neuroscience 10:1051-1069. 11.Voronin LL (1985) In: Buzsaki G, Vanderwolf CH (eds.) Electrical Activity of the Archicortex. Academiai Kiado, Budapest, pp 295-317. 12.Voronin LL, Kuhnt U, Hess G (1987) (submitted).

Plasticity-Related Synaptic Mechanisms in Hippocampus

G. L. COLLINGRIDGE, C. E. HERRON, and R. A. J. LESTER

Department of Pharmacology, University of Bristol, Bristol, BS8 1TD, United Kingdom

The characteristics of NMDA and non-NMDA components of synaptic transmission in the hippocampus have been compared during low frequency transmission in depolarised cells and high frequency transmission under normal conditions. In both cases NMDA receptors mediate a slower rising and longer lasting synaptic response.

NMDA receptors are involved in high frequency transmission (Herron et al, 1986) and the induction of long term potentiation (LTP) (Collingridge et al, 1983) in the Schaffer collateral-commissural pathway in the hippocampus. During low frequency stimulation, however, these receptors do not contribute appreciably to synaptic transmission unless Mg^{2+} is omitted from the perfusate, synaptic inhibition is reduced by a convulsant or the cell under study is greatly depolarised (see Collingridge and Bliss, 1987). We have now further characterised transmission at this synapse under conditions where NMDA receptors mediate a component of the synaptic potential.

Experiments were performed on transverse rat hippocampal slices in the presence of 1 or 2 mM Mg^{2+}. Discontinuous current- and voltage-clamp recordings were obtained from CA1 neurones in response to low (0.033 Hz) or high (100 Hz) frequency stimulation of Schaffer collateral-commissural fibres. The selective antagonist D-2-amino-5-phosphonovalerate (APV, 20 or 50 uM) was used to define the NMDA receptor-mediated synaptic component.

In 7 caesium-loaded cells, examined under voltage-clamp conditions, recordings were obtained at membrane potentials of between -30 and +30 mV, in the presence of 50 uM picrotoxin. In all cells both NMDA and non-NMDA receptor-mediated components were present at all stimulus intensities used. The two components had similar onset latencies and reversal potentials of between 0 and -8 mV. However, the NMDA receptor component had a slower rise-time, longer time to peak and longer duration (Fig 1).

In a separate study, performed under current clamp conditions on 31 cells, with synaptic inhibition unimpaired and at membrane potentials close to rest (-65 to -75 mV) the NMDA receptor component could only be observed when high frequency (> 5 Hz) stimulation was

H. L. Haas G. Buzsàki (Eds.)
Synaptic Plasticity in the Hippocampus
© Springer-Verlag Berlin Heidelberg 1988

employed. Again this component had a slower rise-time, longer time to peak and longer duration than the non-NMDA receptor mediated (ie fast) epsps (Fig 2). However, the NMDA receptor component had a slower latency to onset than the first fast epsp.

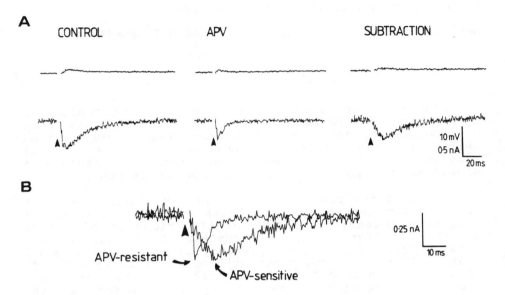

Fig. 1. Partially voltage-clamped response of a CA1 neurone (at -23 mV) to low frequency stimulation, in the presence of picrotoxin. A Averages of 5 successive records showing control, the effect of 20 uM APV and the difference between them. B The non-NMDA (APV-resistant) and NMDA (subtraction) receptor-mediated components are superimposed to emphasise the different time-courses but similar latencies to onset. Arrowheads mark time of stimulus; stimulus artefacts were blanked.

The observation that, in depolarised cells, the onset latencies of both synaptic components were indistinguishable supports the suggestion that neurotransmitter released at a single synapse in the CA1 region of the hippocampus acts upon both NMDA and non-NMDA receptors. Under physiological conditions, however, a single fast epsp does not provide sufficient depolarisation to alleviate appreciably the Mg^{2+} block of NMDA channels (Nowak et al, 1984) since it is rapidly curtailed by synaptic inhibition (Herron et al, 1985; Dingledine et al, 1986). Two or more appropriately timed fast epsps can activate the NMDA receptor system since neurones are maintained for a sufficient duration at membrane potentials where the Mg^{2+} block of NMDA channels is reduced. It would appear therefore that the interplay between synaptic excitation and inhibition is critical in controlling the expression of the NMDA receptor system.

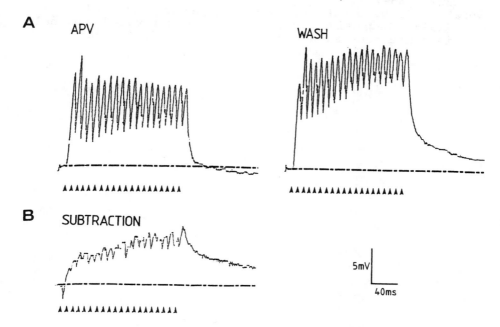

Fig. 2. Responses of a CA1 neurone (at −75 mV) to high frequency (100 Hz, 200 ms) stimulation. A Shows records in the presence and following wash-out of 20 uM APV, respectively. Note that APV had no consistent effect on the fast epsps but reduced an associated depolarisation. B The difference between the records in A showing the NMDA receptor-mediated component.

References

Collingridge GL, Kehl SJ, McLennan H (1983) Excitatory amino acids in synaptic transmission in the Schaffer collateral-commissural pathway of the rat hippocampus. J Physiol (Lond) 334: 33-46

Collingridge GL, Bliss TVP (1987) NMDA receptors - their role in long term potentiation. TINS 10: 288-293

Dingledine R, Hynes M, King GL (1986) Involvement of N-methyl-D-aspartate receptors in epileptiform bursting in the rat hippocampal slice. J Physiol (Lond) 380: 175-189

Herron CE, Williamson R, Collingridge GL (1985) A selective N-methyl-D-aspartate antagonist depresses epileptiform activity in rat hippocampal slices. Neurosci Lett 61: 255-260

Herron CE, Lester RAJ, Coan EJ, Collingridge GL (1986) Frequency-dependent involvement of NMDA receptors in the hippocampus: a novel synaptic mechanism. Nature 322: 265-268

Nowak L, Bregestovski P, Ascher P, Herbet A, Prochiantz A (1984) Magnesium gates glutamate-activated channels in mouse central neurones. Nature 307: 462-465

NMDA Receptor Control of Spontaneous Complex Spike Discharge in Hippocampal Pyramidal Cells

W.C. ABRAHAM and E.W. KAIRISS

Department of Psychology and the Neuroscience Centre, University of Otago,
Dunedin, New Zealand

The NMDA receptor antagonist APV was applied intraventricularly
to determine its effect on the complex spike firing pattern of
spontaneously active hippocampal pyramidal cells. Following APV
delivery complex spike firing decreased by 36% while after saline
injection only a 5% decrease was observed. This effect could not be
explained by changes in firing rate per se but appeared to be related
to the degree of blockade of commissurally induced long-term
potentiation.

Hippocampal pyramidal cells can be induced to fire in bursts in a
variety of ways that appear to involve activation of NMDA receptors.
Not only does iontophoretic application of NMDA elicit bursting (Peet,
Curry, Magnuson & McLennan, 1986) but this and other types of induced
bursting can be blocked by NMDA receptor antagonists such as
2-amino-5-phosphonovalerate (APV; Peet et al., 1986; Hablitz, 1985;
Slater, Stelzer & Galvan, 1985; Herron, Lester, Coan & Collingridge,
1985). In addition, activation of NMDA receptors leads to the
induction of long-term potentiation (LTP), which can also be blocked
by APV (Collingridge, Kehl & McLennan, 1983).

When recorded extracellularly in vivo, hippocampal pyramidal
cells may 'spontaneously' fire in bursts known as complex spikes.
Complex spikes are characterized by varying spike amplitudes and
interspike intervals within the burst that are at least superficially
similar to those same characteristics of APV-sensitive bursts recorded
intracellularly in vitro (Peet et al., 1986). The present study was
designed to determine whether spontaneous complex spiking in vivo is
also sensitive to NMDA receptor antagonists.

Twelve urethane anaesthetised rats were prepared with 30 gauge
cannulae bilaterally in the lateral ventricle, 25 um wire recording
electrodes bilaterally in the cell layer of area CA1, and a single
monopolar stimulating electrode in the ventral hippocampal commissure
near the midline. Recording electrodes were positioned to record
cells showing spontaneous complex spike discharge plus field
potentials evoked by commissural stimulation. Spontaneous unit
activity and field responses evoked by 0.05 Hz test pulses were
recorded throughout the experiment. Saline (5 µl) was injected into
one hemisphere for 10 min followed 10 min later by D,L-APV infusion

H.L. Haas   G. Buzsàki (Eds.)
Synaptic Plasticity in the Hippocampus
© Springer-Verlag Berlin Heidelberg 1988

(40-80 mM, pH 7.0, 5 µl, for 10 min) into the other. Unit activity was selected via a window discriminator, sampled by the computer and analysed in 5 min epochs: just prior to injections, plus 5-10 min, 40-45 min and 90-95 min after APV infusion. High-frequency trains were applied to the commissure to induce LTP at 50 min following APV.

Twenty units, divided equally among the two groups, were successfully recorded throughout the recording session. Forty min after APV delivery, the number of spikes per burst was reduced in 7/10 cells from 3.2 to 2.5 (a mean reduction of 36% assuming that a reduction to 1 spike represents complete burst abolition). No reduction was apparent 5 min after injection and the reduction was still 31% after 90 min. Saline administration did not result in any significant change in the number of spikes per burst at any time period, the maximal reduction being 5% at the 40 and 90 min intervals. Trains were delivered and LTP induced 50 min following APV injection, but this did alter the pattern of bursting for either group (compare the 40 and 90 min results). Three cells in the APV group were not included in the analysis since large LTP of equivalent magnitude to that generated contralaterally (saline side), was elicited in these hemispheres. We assumed that this reflected a poor penetration of the APV into CA1, perhaps due to placement of the cannulae outside the ventricular system. These cells showed a mean increase in spikes per burst of 27% after 40 min that returned to a mere 4% increase by the 90 min interval.

In three animals for which bilateral unit activity data was available, the field potentials were suitably matched to permit a comparison of within-animal drug effects on unit activity and commissurally evoked LTP. At 40 min after APV delivery (10 min prior to tetanisation), these animals had reductions in spikes per burst in the APV treated hemisphere of 18%, 57% and 62%. The corresponding reductions in LTP were 8%, 45% and 78%, with a correlation between the two variables of 0.92. We interpret these data as indicating that a single effect of APV, i.e. a partial block of NMDA receptors, is mediating both of the observed effects.

An analysis of the number of firing episodes per epoch showed a slow steady decline over time that was essentially equivalent between the two hemispheres. This rules out the possibility that the altered spiking in the APV group was secondary to a change in some factor governing the cell's firing rate, e.g. a simple reduction in the rate of afferent activity or an elevated action potential threshold. However it is not possible with intraventricular administration to determine the site of action of the applied drug. APV clearly penetrated the recording area since LTP was affected there, but the effect on unit activity could have been mediated by an altered pattern of afferent activity. This issue will require additional study using local microinjections or iontophoresis.

The data presented above clearly indicate that APV alters complex spike discharge in CA1 pyramidal cells by reducing the number of spikes per burst. The functional significance of complex spike discharge is not known, although it appears to be a normal mode of firing since it can be observed in cells which are recorded for days at a time (P.J. Best, personal communication). If this spontaneous bursting is in fact due to activation of NMDA receptors, then these receptors may have a relatively low threshold for activation in vivo. By implication, LTP may also have a lower threshold and be more likely to occur normally than one might have predicted from the train strength required to induce it experimentally. While the duration of a single burst (usually <20 ms) is unlikely to be sufficiently long to induce LTP, rapidly repeated complex spike discharge (e.g. when the animal is in the cell's place field, cf. O'Keefe, 1979) may then be sufficient to reach LTP threshold. Finally it should be noted that the altered complex spike discharge represents an effect of APV that is additional to its effect on LTP. Therefore effects of the drug on behaviour might be caused by alterations in either LTP or the neuronal signalling that normally includes burst firing. Separation of these confounded effects may not be a simple matter.

Supported by the New Zealand Medical Research Council.

REFERENCES

Collingridge, G.L., Kehl, S.J. & McLennan, H. _J. Physiol_. 1983, 334: 33-46.

Hablitz, J.J. _Cell. Mol. Neurobiol_. 1985, 5: 389-405.

Herron, C.E., Lester, R.A.J., Coan, E.J. & Collingridge, G.L. _Neurosci. Lett_. 1985, 60: 19-23.

O'Keefe, J.O. _Prog. Neurobiol_. 1979, 13: 419-439.

Peet, M.J., Curry, K., Magnuson, D.S. & McLennan, H. _Can. J. Physiol. Pharmacol_. 1986, 64: 163-168.

Slater, N.T., Stelzer, A. & Galvan, M. _Neurosci. Lett_. 1985, 60: 25-31.

Mecamylamine Blocks Responses to NMDA and a Component of Synaptic Transmission in Rat Hippocampal Slices

J. F. Blake, M. W. Brown, N. Al-Ani[1], E. J. Coan[1], and G. L. Collingridge[1]

Departments of Anatomy and Pharmacology[1], University of Bristol, Bristol, BS8 1TD, United Kingdom

The effects of the ganglionic nicotinic antagonist mecamylamine have been determined on amino acid- and synaptically-evoked responses in rat hippocampal slices. Mecamylamine selectively blocked responses mediated by NMDA receptors.

Activation of the N-methyl-D-aspartate (NMDA) receptor system is required for the induction of long term potentiation (LTP) in the Schaffer collateral-commissural pathway (Collingridge et al, 1983). Consequently, drugs which depress this receptor system would be predicted to impair this form of synaptic plasticity and any associated cognitive function.

Mecamylamine is a ganglionic, nicotinic antagonist. There is reason to believe, however, that it may also be an excitatory amino acid antagonist, since it was found to reduce the excitation of nigral neurones by L-aspartic acid (GLC, unpublished observations) and of motoneurones by L-glutamate (Evans, 1978). In the present study, therefore, we have examined the effects of mecamylamine on acidic amino acid-induced and synaptically-evoked responses in the hippocampus.

Experiments were performed on transverse rat hippocampal slices, which were perfused ($1-2$ ml min^{-1}) initially with 1 mM Mg^{2+}-containing medium followed by Mg^{2+}-free medium. To determine the effects of mecamylamine on agonist-induced responses, slices were set up for grease-gap recording from the alveus, as described previously (Blake et al, 1986). In 3 slices in Mg^{2+}-free medium, mecamylamine (100 uM, 90 min) reduced reversibly responses induced by 5-20 uM NMDA, but had little effect on responses induced by 20 uM quisqualate (QA) or 5 uM $\propto$-amino-3-hydroxy-5-methyl-4-isoazole-propionic acid (AMPA) (Fig. 1.).

To examine the effects of mecamylamine on synaptic potentials, microelectrode recordings of field potentials were obtained from the CA1 cell body region in response to 0.08 Hz stimulation of the Schaffer collateral-commissural pathway. In Mg^{2+}-free medium, secondary population spikes, mediated by activation of NMDA receptors (Coan and Collingridge, 1985), can be recorded.

H. L. Haas G. Buzsàki (Eds.)
Synaptic Plasticity in the Hippocampus
© Springer-Verlag Berlin Heidelberg 1988

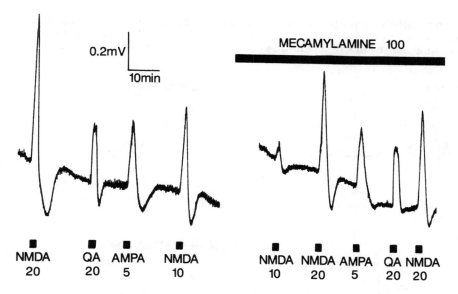

Fig. 1. The effects of mecamylamine on depolarisations of CA1 neurones induced by acidic amino acids. Agonists were applied in 2 ml volumes. The first agonist response in mecamylamine was obtained after 30 min of perfusion of the antagonist. Concentrations are given in uM.

Mecamylamine (100 uM) substantially reduced or eliminated these secondary population spikes, in all 10 slices studied. The time course of antagonism was relatively slow; frequently taking up to 90-120 min to achieve maximum effect and greater than 60-120 min of washing for full recovery. This contrasted to the competitive NMDA antagonist D-2-amino-5-phosphonovalerate (20 uM; APV) which, when tested on the same slices, was fully effective within 10 min and totally reversible after a 20-30 min wash. At 10 uM, mecamylamine also reduced the secondary population spikes in all 3 slices examined (Fig. 2.). In contrast to mecamylamine, hexamethonium (250 uM, 90 min) had little effect on the synaptic response in 6 slices, suggesting that nicotinic receptors were not involved.

These data indicate that mecamylamine is an NMDA antagonist. It can therefore be added to the growing list of secondary and tertiary amines which are also NMDA antagonists. Others include chlorpromazine and diazepam (Evans et al, 1977), ketamine and phencyclidine (Anis et al, 1983) and MK-801 (Wong et al, 1986). These compounds may all act in a similar manner, such as by blocking the NMDA channel.

Mecamylamine administered systemically can penetrate into the brain. It is possible, therefore, that actions at the NMDA receptor system may contribute to certain central effects, such as confusion and hallucinations, that are seen when high doses of this drug are given.

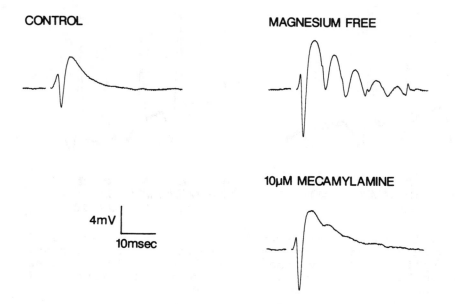

Fig. 2. The effects of mecamylamine on synaptic responses. Representative single records to illustrate the response in 1_2 mM Mg^{2+} (control), 30 min following perfusion with Mg^{2+}-free medium and 120 min after the addition of mecamylamine to the Mg^{2+}-free perfusate. Stimulus artefacts have been blanked.

References

Anis NA, Berry SC, Burton NR, Lodge D (1983) The dissociative anaesthetics, ketamine and phencyclidine, selectively reduce excitation of central mammalian neurones by N-methyl-aspartate. Br J Pharmac 79: 565-575

Blake JF, Brown MW, Collingridge GL, Evans RH (1986) Simple measurement of amino acid-induced polarization of hippocampal CA1 pyramidal neurones in vitro. Br J Pharmac 88: 273P

Coan EJ, Collingridge GL (1985) Magnesium ions block an N-methyl-D-aspartate receptor-mediated component of synaptic transmission in rat hippocampus. Neurosci Lett 53: 21-26

Collingridge GL, Kehl SJ, McLennan H (1983) Excitatory amino acids in synaptic transmission in the Schaffer collateral-commissural pathway of the rat hippocampus. J Physiol (Lond) 334: 33-46

Evans RH (1978) Cholinoceptive properties of motoneurones of the immature rat spinal cord maintained in vitro. Neuropharmacology 17: 277-279

Evans RH, Francis AA, Watkins JC (1977) Differential antagonism by chlorpromazine and diazepam of frog motoneurone depolarization induced by glutamate-related amino acids. Eur J Pharmac 44: 325-330

Wong EHF, Kemp JA, Priestley T, Knight AR, Woodruff GN, Iversen LL (1986) The anticonvulsant MK-801 is a potent N-methyl-D-aspartate antagonist. Proc Natl Acad Sci USA 83: 7104-7108

Long-Term Potentiation in the Recurrent Inhibitory Circuit of the Dentate Gyrus

M. L. ERRINGTON[1], H. L. HAAS[2], and T. V. P. BLISS[1]

[1] National Institute for Medical Research, Mill Hill, London NW7 1AA and
[2] Department of Physiology, University of Mainz, 6500 Mainz, Federal Republic of Germany

Evidence obtained from intracellular and field potential recordings demonstrates that the circuit mediating recurrent inhibition in the dentate gyrus is capable of sustaining long-term potentiation following high-frequency antidromic stimulation of mossy fibres.

The question of whether long-term potentiation occurs in the inhibitory circuits of the hippocampus remains controversial. Buszaki and Eidelberg (1982), recording extracellularly from putative interneurones (basket cells) in the dentate gyrus and area CA1 of the anaesthetized rat, found a prolonged increase in probability of cell firing to afferent stimulation after high-frequency stimulation of Schaffer-commissural fibres, and concluded that LTP occurs at excitatory feedforward synapses onto interneurones. Similarly, Kairis et al (1987) have presented field potential evidence for LTP in feedforward synapses onto inhibitory neurones in the dentate gyrus of the anaesthetized rat. In the hippocampal slice, on the other hand, the available evidence suggests that LTP of feedforward synapses does not occur in area CA1 (Yamamoto and Chujo, 1978; Misgeld et al., 1979; Haas and Rose, 1982; Griffith et al., 1986; Abraham et al., 1987). In this paper we present in vivo and in vitro evidence that LTP occurs in the circuit mediating recurrent inhibition in the dentate gyrus.

In vivo experiments were performed on adult male Spague-Dawley rats anaesthetized with urethane (1.5 g/kg, i.p.). Stimulating electrodes were placed in the angular bundle to activate the perforant path and in the hilus to activate mossy fibres, with recording electrodes in the granule cell and CA3 pyramidal cell layers, as indicated in Fig. 1. The recurrent inhibitory circuit in the dentate gyrus was activated by conditioning shocks delivered to the mossy fibres, leading to antidromic invasion of granule cells. The degree of inhibition was assessed by the reduction in the population spike evoked by test shocks given to the perforant path, with the conditioning-test interval adjusted to be optimal for each animal. Inhibition curves, expressing the amplitude of the orthodromic test spike as a function of the amplitude of the antidromic conditioning spike, were constructed before and 30-50 min after a high-frequency train (250 Hz for 200 msec), sufficient to induce LTP in the mossy fibre pathway to CA3, was delivered to the mossy fibre electrode. To ensure that the granule cells activated by the mossy fibre electrode overlapped at least partially with the population activated by the perforant path electrode, shocks were given via both electrodes separately and again nearly simultaneously; only those electrode placements were accepted in which the algebraic sum of the antidromic and orthodromic spikes was greater than the spike evoked by near-simultaneous activation. In 4/4 such

H.L. Haas   G. Buzsàki (Eds.)
Synaptic Plasticity in the Hippocampus
© Springer-Verlag Berlin Heidelberg 1988

experiments the inhibition curve was shifted to the left after tetanic stimulation of the mossy fibres, indicating a prolonged enhancement of inhibition (Fig 2).

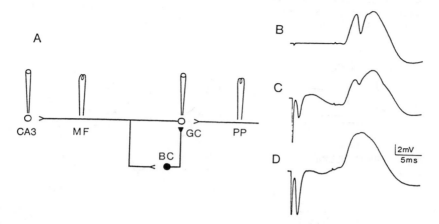

FIG. 1. A. Arrangement of stimulating and recording electrodes for in vivo experiments. B-D. Responses evoked in the granule cell layer by a test shock to the perforant path (B), and the graded inhibition of the orthodromic population spike by preceding antidromic stimulation (C,D). (MF mossy fibres, GC granule cell, BC basket cell, PP perforant path).

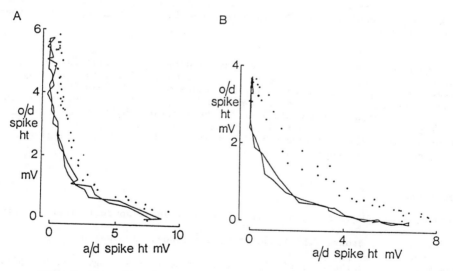

FIG. 2. Two examples of LTP in the recurrent inhibitory circuit of the dentate gyrus. Test shocks to the perforant path were preceded at a fixed, optimal interval (8-15 msec) by a series of antidromic stimuli of varying strengths. The amplitude of the orthodromic population spike is plotted as a function of the amplitude of the preceding antidromic spike before (dots) and 30-50 min after (lines) a tetanus to the mossy fibres. Note the leftward shift of the inhibition curve induced by the tetanus.

The effects of high-frequency stimulation of mossy fibres on inhibitory potentials recorded from granule cells with intracellular electrodes was examined in the hippocampal slice preparation. With KCl electrodes a bicucculine-sensitive depolarizing inhibitory potential was obtained which in some cases was able to fire the cell (Fig 3B), and which could be potentiated by mossy fibre tetanization (Fig 3C).

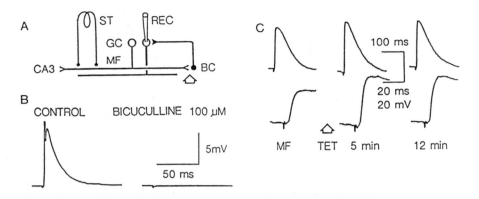

FIG. 3. LTP at the granule cell-basket cell synapse in vitro. A. Arrangement of electrodes. B,C. Intracellular recordings (averages of 8 sweeps) from granule cells with KCl filled electrodes reveals a depolarizing potential (ipsp) following mossy fibre stimulation. B. The ipsp can fire action potentials (clipped in B, control), and is completely blocked by bicucculine. C. The ipsp is potentiated by tetanic stimulation of mossy fibres.

Although these results indicate that recurrent inhibition in the dentate gyrus can be potentiated by high-frequency stimulation of mossy fibres, it is not clear which of the two limbs of the disynaptic circuit (mossy fibre collateral to basket cell, or basket cell to granule cell) is potentiated - either case would lead to the leftward shift of the inhibition curve, and potentiation of the granule cell recurrent inhibitory potential. A resolution of this question will require direct recording from interneurones.

REFERENCES

Abraham, W.C., Gustafsson, B. & Wigstrom, H. (1987). Journal of Physiology, In press.
Griffith, W.H., Brown, T.H. & Johnston, D. (1986). Journal of Neurophysiology, 35, 767-775.
Buzsaki, G. & Eidelberg E. (1982) Journal of Neurophysiology, 48, 597-607.
Haas, H.L. & Rose, G. (1982). Journal of Physiology, 329, 541-552.
Kairiss, E., Abraham, W.C., Bilkey, D.K. & Goddard, G.V. (1987). Brain Research, 401, 87-95.
Misgeld, U., Sarvey, J.M., & Klee, M.R. (1979). Experimental Brain Research, 59, 217-229.
Yamamoto, C. & Chujo, T. (1978). Experimental Neurology, 58, 242-250.

NMDA Receptors May Be Involved in Generation of Hippocampal Theta Rhythm

Z. Horváth, A. Kamondi, J. Czopf, T. V. P. Bliss[1], and G. Buzsàki

Department of Physiology, Medical School, Pécs, Hungary, and [1]MRC Unit, London, United Kingdom

Male rats were implanted with chronic recording electrodes in the hippocampus and dentate gyrus and injection cannulae in the lateral ventricles. EEG was recorded while the rat was running in a wheel for water reward and power density spectra were calculated.

Neither atropine (50 mg/kg, i.p.) nor 2-APV (5 ul, 2%; intra-ventricular) alone was able to abolish hippocampal theta waves during running. However, when the drugs were given together, theta EEG was replaced by irregular activity and no peaks were present in the 5-10 Hz band of the power spectrum. Similarly, when atropine and CPP (40 mg/kg, i.p.) were given separately theta activity survived but rhythmicity was completely absent when the drugs were given together. Vanderwolf and Leung (1983) reported similar findings with a combination of phencyclidine and atropine earlier.

These findings suggest that NMDA receptors are involved in mediating the atropine-resistant form of theta EEG in the hippocampus.

Vanderwolf CH and Leung LS (1983) In W. Seifert (ed.), Molecular, Cellular and Behavioral Neurobiology of the Hippocampus, Academic Press, New York.

H.L. Haas   G. Buzsàki (Eds.)
Synaptic Plasticity in the Hippocampus
© Springer-Verlag Berlin Heidelberg 1988

Cytoplasmic Ca^{2+} Changes in Reference to Long-Term Potentiation in the Hippocampal Slice

H. Kato, K. Ito, H. Miyakawa, A. Ogura[1], and Y. Kudo

Department of Physiology Yamagata University Medical School, Yamagata and
[1]Department Neuroscience Mitsubishi-Kasei Institute of Life Sciences, Machida-Shi, Tokyo, Japan

Microfluorometry of the guinea-pig hippocampal slice loaded with Ca^{2+}-indicator was carried out in parallel with extracellular population spike recording. Increase of the fluorescence, most probably representing elevation of Ca^{2+} level in postsynaptic cytoplasm of CA1 pyramidal cells, occurred upon establishment of LTP. However, exposure to high K medium or NMDA which did not lead to LTP also evoked comparable fluorescence increase.

We have recently established a video-assisted microfluorometry system using fura-2 as a Ca^{2+}-indicator, which enables a real-time multi-site determination of cytoplasmic Ca^{2+} concentration ($[Ca^{2+}]_i$). This is applicable not only to isolated hippocampal neurons under culture (1,2) but to brain slice preparations (3). Examinations on the cultured neurons revealed that the $[Ca^{2+}]_i$ in the resting state was around 50 nM and that an activation of L-glutamate receptor by its agonists elevated the $[Ca^{2+}]_i$ to around 1 µM. Similar fluorescence rises were observed in the somatic and dendritic layers of granule cells in the guinea-pig dentate gyrus when perforant path was tetanically stimulated. Since these were significantly slow in rising phase, long-lasting in decay phase and blocked reversibly by a receptor blocker (2-aminophosphonovalerate) we concluded that the fluorescence rises represented the elevation of $[Ca^{2+}]_i$ of postsynaptic cytoplasm of the granule cells rather than that of presynaptic cytosol of the perforant path terminals. Here, the CA1 region of hippocampal slice was subjected to the identical fluorometry.

Hippocampal slices (300 µm thick) were prepared with a rotary cutter within 5 min after sacrifice. Loading of the indicator was done by soaking twice the slice in normal Krebs solution containing 5 µM fura-2 acetoxymethylester for 30 min each. This might cause an excess loading of the dye, but otherwise unneglibly strong autofluorescence of the slice interfered with the signal of fura-2. The slice was then placed on a thin glass coverslip mounted on an epifluorescence microscope and was illuminated by ultraviolet beams of 340 nm and 380 nm wavelengths alternately. The image was displayed on a CRT by the aid of an SIT video-camera. The brightness of the CRT image, proportionated to the fluorescence intensity, was measured by an array of photodiodes. Ratio of fluorescence intensities under two excitation wavelengths coming in neighbor was continuously calculated (F_{340}/F_{380}) by a desk-top computer.

H.L. Haas   G. Buzsàki (Eds.)
Synaptic Plasticity in the Hippocampus
© Springer-Verlag Berlin Heidelberg 1988

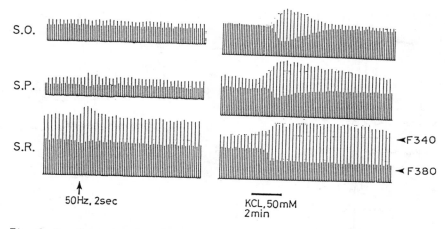

Fig. 1. Sample traces of fluorescence recording from three representative sites. Note increases of fluorescence under 340 nm
beam (F_{340}) and decreases of that under 380 nm (F_{380}) upon
stimulations. Note also variation in the absolute fluorescence
intensities between layers.

A glass capillary electrode was placed in the stratum pyramidale of CA1 region under the fluorescence measurement, through
which monitored were the amplitudes of population spikes evoked
by Schaeffer collateral stimuli delivered at regular intervals
via a tungsten bipolar electrode.

The slice was exposed to a continuous perfusion of oxygenated Krebs solution (35°C). NMDA was included in this medium.
Elevation of KCl concentration was done by equimolar replacement
of NaCl in the medium.

Fluorescence intensity was not equal among the layers of CA1
region; dim in stratum pyramidale (S.P.), bright in strata oriens
(S.O.) and radiatum (S.R.). This was due both to the amount of
fura-2 loaded (S.P. < S.O. < S.R.) and to local variation of
$[Ca^{2+}]_i$ as indicated by the F_{340}/F_{380} values (S.O. < S.P. < S.R.;
Fig. 1).

As shown in Fig. 2, the F_{340}/F_{380} values of all layers
elevated when Schaeffer pathway was tetanically stimulated (500
µA, 0.2 ms, 50 Hz, 2 s). But the amplitudes of the elevation
varied between layers (S.O. < S.P. < S.R.). In this and other
samples, similar pattern of F_{340}/F_{380}-elevation was evoked when
LTP was established by the Schaeffer stimulation.

The exposure to 50 mM K⁺-containing medium also induced elevation of the F_{340}/F_{380} values. Note that LTP was not evoked in
this case, although the amplitude of the elevation was even
larger than that in the case of Schaeffer stimulation.

The application of 100 µM NMDA induced a layer-dependent
elevation of the F_{340}/F_{380} value (Fig. 3). But LTP was never
established by this protocol of stimulation.

Still we are devoid of superfluous evidence that the observed elevation in the fluorescence ratio exclusively represented
the rise of $[Ca^{2+}]_i$ in the postsynaptic cytoplasm. But if we

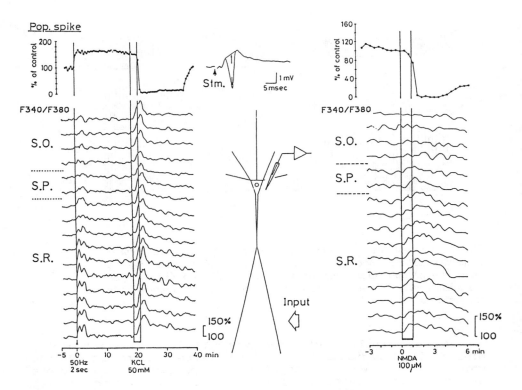

Fig. 2. *Sample of simultaneous recordings of population spike and fluorescence. Pre-stimulus values of spike amplitude and F_{340}/F_{380} were taken as 100 %. Note that Schaeffer stimulation induced LTP, while KCl stimulation did not even after a transient synaptic suppression was over. Here the recording was truncated for saving space. Single KCl exposures never induced LTP in this and other trials.*

Fig. 3. *Case of NMDA application. Single NMDA exposures failed to induce LTP in this and other trials.*

assume so, we could expect that the $[Ca^{2+}]_i$-elevation would be accompanied by the establishment of LTP, as suggested by the theory of receptor number increase due to activation of Ca^{2+}-dependent protease (4). The present results, especially those of K^+- and NMDA-stimulation failed to support it. We do not say that $[Ca^{2+}]_i$ is independent of LTP, since the electrically evoked LTP was always accompanied by the elevation of F_{340}/F_{380} values. The view favorable at present is that $[Ca^{2+}]_i$ might not be a sole factor for the establishment of LTP.

References

1. *Y. Kudo & A. Ogura, Br. J. Pharmacol.,* __89__, *191, '86.*
2. *A. Ogura, T. Iijima & Y. Kudo, Neurosci. Lett.,* *in press.*
3. *Y. Kudo et al., Brain Res.,* __407__, *168, '87.*
4. *G. Lynch & M. Baudry, Science,* __224__, *1057, '84.*

Electron Histochemical Localization of Calcium in CA1 of Hippocampal Slices Following High Frequency Stimulation: Effects of Excitatory Amino Acid Antagonists

L. Siklos[1], U. Kuhnt[2], F. Joo[1], and A. Mihaly[1]

[1]Institute of Biophysics, Biological Research Center, 6701 Szeged, Hungary
[2]Max-Planck-Institut für Biophysikalische Chemie, 3400 Göttingen, Federal Republic of Germany
[3]Department of Anatomy, University Medical School, 6701 Szeged, Hungary

Summary: Experiments were performed to localize calcium in CA1 of hippocampal slices (i) under control condition, (ii) after generation of LTP, (iii) after blockade of LTP by APV, and (iiii) after blockade of synaptic transmission by GDEE. The physiological experiments were followed by immersion fixation in modified Winborn fixative and the pattern of Ca-containing deposits was investigated. The dendritic deposits were restricted to a sublamina of str.radiatum. The highest density of dendritic deposits was found 280-350 μm distal to the str.pyramidale. The location of this sublamina correlated with the position of the stimulating electrode.

In an earlier study we have shown with histochemical techniques that membrane bound Ca is increased during long-term potentiation (LTP) (1). The number of electron dense deposits (EDD) containing Ca (3) was significantly increased following the generation of LTP, both at the pre- and the postsynaptic site. In the present study we have investigated the effect of two excitatory amino acid receptor antagonists on the distribution of Ca containing EDDs in mitochondria after high frequency stimulation. Glutamic acid diethyl ester (GDEE), a relatively unspecific antagonist was used in a concentration which totally blocked synaptic transmission, and 5-amino-phosphono valeric acid (a highly specific antagonist of the N-methyl-D-aspartate receptor) was used in a concentration which blocked LTP. Both antagonists diminished the number of EDDs in mitochondria on the pre- and postsynaptic site.

Transverse hippocampal slices (500 μm) were prepared from the right hippocampus of adult guinea pigs. Slices were kept in a storage chamber at room temperature and later on transferred to the recording chamber. The perfusion medium had the following composition (mM): 124 NaCl, 5 KCl, 1.25 NaH_2PO_4, 2.0 $MgSO_4$, 2.0 $CaCl_2$, 26 $NaHCO_3$, and 10 glucose, it was saturated with O_2/CO_2 (95/5%). Recordings were performed at 35±1°C. Monopolar stimulating electrodes were placed in str.rad. of CA3 near the border of CA3/CA1 and in str.or.; recording electrodes were positioned in str.pyr. and str.rad. of CA1. During the control periods both pathways were stimulated intermittently at 0.25/s. High frequency stimulation was given to Schaffer Collaterals/Commissural pathway only; the trains consisted of 20 stimuli at 100 Hz. The train was repeated 5 times at

H.L. Haas   G. Buzsàki (Eds.)
Synaptic Plasticity in the Hippocampus
© Springer-Verlag Berlin Heidelberg 1988

intervals of 8s. APV (100 μM) and GDEE (20 mM) were applied via the medium 30 min before the tetanic stimulation and switched off 5 min thereafter. In 'control' slices no tetanic trains were given, but only low frequency stimulation over the total recording period (2-3h). Two hours after tetanic stimulation slices were transferred to the cold fixative solution which contained 10 mM $CaCl_2$. After fixaton for two days, the regio superior was cut out, fixed for additional 3 h, osmicated for 2h at 4°C and conventionally processed for electron microscopy. Ultrathin sections (stained with lead citrate only) were examined on either a Zeiss EM10 or a Jeol 100B electron microscope. A method was developed to determine the spatial distribution of Ca-containing EDDs by directly attaching a X/Y-plotter to the EM (4). The specimen moving knobs of the EM were fitted with potentiometers and the signals from them were directly fed to the inputs of the X/Y-recorder. Thus the position of the recorder pen correlated with sample points. By using this 'electron microscopic camera lucida', firstly the outline of the section and secondly the central line of str.pyr. were drawn. Thereafter, sections were systematically traced for Ca-containing EDDs. Only mitochondria, which contained one or more round shaped deposits were counted and marked at their appropriate position on the X/Y-recorder.

Mitochondria containing EDDs were found in axons and in dendrites. They were classified and counted according to their location. In GDEE treated slices dendritic EDDs were only seen occasionaly or not at all (Fig.1A). Under all the other experimental and control conditions, EDDs containing mitochondria were clustered in a stripe 280-350 μm distally from the pyramidal cell layer (Fig.1B-

Fig.1 *Localization and density distribution of Ca-containing mitochondria.*

On the left side is shown the investigated area of ultrathin sections and the location of EDD containing mitochondria. Orientation as indicated, calibration bar is 100 μm. EDD containing mitochondria are marked (full circles: dendritic localization; open circles: axonal localization). Right side: density distribution of EDD containing mitochondria along the axis of the pyramidal neurones. Open circle, continuous line: dendritic localization. Full circle, broken line: axonal localization. A) GDEE treatment (20 mM): no dendritic deposits are seen. Axonal deposits (n=95) are distributed over str.rad.. Measured area: 229080 μm². B) Stimulated control: dendritic deposits (n=15) are clustered in a stripe, axonal deposits (n=59) are distributed over str.rad.. Measured area: 244000 μm². C) APV treatment (100 μM): as in (B) dendritic deposits (n=50) are clustered in a stripe. Axonal deposits (n=103) are disturbed over str.rad.. Measured area: 249660 μm². D) Successful induction of LTP: dendritic deposits (n=73) are clustered in a sublamina in str.rad.. Axonal deposits (n=246) are spread over str.rad.. Measured area: 263370 μm².

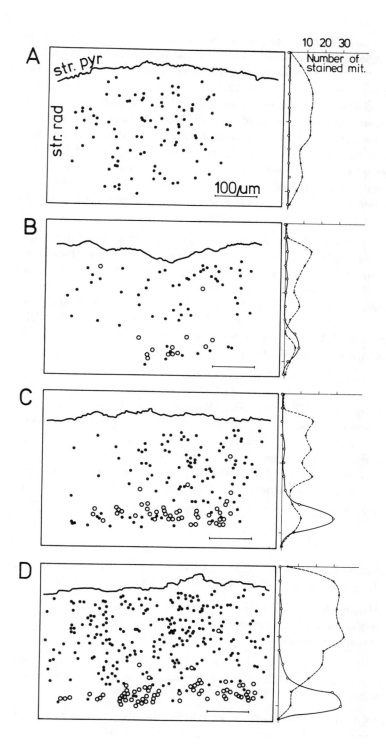

D). The highest concentration was seen in slices in which LTP was successfully generated. APV treated material showed a substantial reduction of EDDs when compared with LTP slices. Stimulated control slices displayed even less EDD loaded mitochondria in dendrites. The localization of these mitochondria roughly coincided with the position of the stimulating electrode in str.rad.. In contrast to the sublaminar-restricted distribution of dendritic EDDs, axonal mitochondria containing EDDs were spread at an even density over the total area of str.rad. which was subjected to the analysis. The highest density was observed in LTP-slices; in APV treated slices the density was reduced. As was the case with the dendritic localization, GDEE treated slices displayed the lowest density (Fig.1A-D). The total number of mitochonria (EDD containing and empty mitochondria) did not variy significantly in the slices subjected to analysis.

The distribution of the axonal deposits was unexpected and at present we are unable to give a meaningful interpretation. The dependance of the amount of deposits on the different treatments was also unexpected, particularly because they were present 2h after the tetanic stimulation and thus do not reflect transient changes. More experiments will be necessary to explain these findings. The results concerning the dendritic localization of EDDs containing mitochondria support earlier findings (1,2), in so far as the Ca containing mitochondria are restricted to an area in which the activated fibres presumably contact the dendrites.

In APV treated slices the amount of EDDs is reduced. Nevertheless, compared with stimulated control slices, the amount of EDDs is significantly higher. Judging from the electrical recording, LTP was clearly blocked under this condition. The present results therefore suggest that Ca influxes, which are triggered by tetanic stimulation lead to longer lasting changes of the Ca-binding capacity of mitochondria. However, only the Ca-influx across the Ca channel which is coupled to the NMDA receptor can generate LTP. A selective blockage of the different Ca channels combined with an electron histochemical analysis of Ca deposits might lead to a better understanding of the role of Ca for the generation and maintenance of LTP.

1. U.Kuhnt, A.Mihaly, F.Joo: Increased binding of calcium in the hippocampal. slice during long-term potentiation. Neuroscience Lett., 53 (1985) 149-154

2. U.Kuhnt, A.Mihaly, F.Joo, L.Siklos: Localization of calcium in long-term potentiated CA1 region of the hippocampal slice: a combined electrophysiological and histochemical study. Submitted

3. A.Mihaly, U.Kuhnt, F.Joo, L.Siklos: Semi-quantitative evaluation of histochemically detectable calcium binding in mammalian brain slices. J.Neurosc. Meth., 20 (1987), 283-293

4. L.Siklos, F.Joo, U.Kuhnt: Method for visualizing the spatial distribution of histochemical precipitates of large areas at the EM-level. Submitted

Transmitter Mechanisms
of Long-Term Potentiation

Involvement of Serotonin in Hippocampal Plasticity

M. Segal and G. Richter

Center for Neurosciences, The Weizmann Institute of Science, Rehovot 76100, Israel

Serotonin (5-hydroxytryptamine, 5-HT) containing fibers originate in the brainstem raphe nuclei and innervate extensively the hippocampus. This innervation is reported to modulate hippocampal reactivity to afferent stimulation in the freely moving rat (Winson 1980) and to affect the expression of long term potentiation of responses to perforant path stimulation (Bliss et al 1983). More recently serotonin has been implicated in the generation of rhythmic hippocampal activity and in "learning" and "memory" (Vanderwolf 1987).

At the cellular level serotonin acts primarily on 5-HT-1A receptors to activate a potassium conductance and hyperpolarize neurons recorded in a slice (Segal 1980). The site of action and the mechanisms underlying the diverse relations of serotonin to the hippocampus behavior remained unclear partly because of the diffuse and apparently nonspecific nature of this innervation. We used the intact anaesthetized rat as well as the brain slice preparation in an attempt to relate the cellular action of serotonin to its gross physiological action. We restricted the serotonergic innervation of the forebrain to the hippocampus by destroying it with specific neurotoxins and implantation of serotonin containing raphe neurons directly into the hippocampus. We then activated the serotonergic innervation of the hippocampus by electrical stimulation (in the slice) or by application of drugs which cause release of serotonin (in the intact brain) and monitored changes in hippocampal functions.

We found that serotonin releasers (e.g. fenfluramine) increase dentate gyrus population spike response to perforant path stimulation. This effect is nearly absent in rats depleted of their serotonin stores but is present in such rats after they were implanted with serotonin containing neurons. This indicates that serotonin acts in the hippocampus proper to enhance reactivity to afferent stimulation. We were able to confirm earlier reports by Bliss et al indicating that serotonin-depleted rats are less capable of maintaining potentiated perforant path responses. This ability could be restored in some rats by grafts of raphe tissue. At the cellular level we found that the grafted serotonin neurons possess identifying physiological properties and make viable connections with the host hippocampus (Segal and Azmitia 1986). Taken together these experiments indicate that the serotonergic effects observed in the hippocampus are indeed exerted at the level of the dentate gyrus and not on regions afferent to this structure. The relations between cellular activity of serotonin neurons,

H. L. Haas   G. Buzsàki (Eds.)
Synaptic Plasticity in the Hippocampus
© Springer-Verlag Berlin Heidelberg 1988

cellular effects of serotonin and behavioral consequences of serotonin activation are currently being investigated.

References

Bliss, T.V.P., Goddard, G.V. and Riives, M. Reduction of long term potentiation in the dentate gyrus of the rat following selective depletion of monoamines. J. Physiol. 1983. 334: 475-491.

Vanderwolf, C.H. Near-total loss of 'learning' and 'memory' as a result of combined cholinergic and serotonergic blockade in the rat. Behav. Brain Res. 1987. 23: 43-45.

Winson, J. Influence of raphe nuclei on neuronal transmission from perforant pathway through dentate gyrus. J. Neurophysiol. 1980. 44: 937-950.

Segal, M. The action of serotonin in the hippocampal slice preparation. J. Physiol. 1980. 33: 423-439.

Segal, M. and Azmitia, E.C. Fetal raphe neurons grafted into the hippocampus develop normal adult physiological properties. Brain Res. 1986. 364: 162-166.

Norepinephrine Enhances Long-Term Potentiation at Hippocampal Mossy Fiber Synapses

D. Johnston, W. F. Hopkins, and R. Gray

Program in Neuroscience, Baylor College of Medicine, Houston, TX 77030, USA

Mossy fiber synapses have a number of relatively unique features, one of which relates to the finding that long-term potentiation (LTP) at these synapses is not dependent on NMDA receptors (1). Norepinephrine (NE), through beta-adrenoceptors, can increase the magnitude, duration, and probability of induction of LTP at mossy fiber synapses. Results of experiments in which we injected cAMP analogs into the postsynaptic neuron and others in which we recorded the activity of single calcium channels suggest that the NE enhancement of LTP takes place postsynaptically through increased calcium influx.

Hippocampal mossy fibers have large and ultrastructurally identifiable synaptic endings, which have been shown to terminate on portions of dendrites that are anatomically and electrotonically proximal to the somata of CA3 pyramidal neurons. The short electrotonic distance of the subsynaptic membrane from the usual somatic recording site has permitted the use of voltage clamp techniques to measure some of the biophysical properties of this synaptic input (2,3). Some of the features of LTP at this synapse have also been recently described (4,5), including the preliminary finding that NE can enhance LTP in a frequency- or activity-dependent manner (6). We have explored further the mechanisms associated with this NE enhancement of LTP at mossy fiber synapses (7). We have also found that NE increases the activity of calcium channels in hippocampal neurons, an action that may underlie the NE modulation of LTP (8).

For the LTP experiments, standard in vitro slice techniques were employed, including extra- and intracellular recordings and single electrode voltage clamping. For the single channel experiments, we utilized an exposed-slice technique in which patch clamping can be performed on adult hippocampal neurons (9).

NE (10 uM) and the beta-adrenoceptor agonist isoproterenol (ISO) (1 uM) had little, if any, effect on excitatory synaptic responses when the mossy fibers were stimulated at low frequency (0.2 Hz), but, when present during a high-frequency stimulus train, increased the magnitude, duration, and probability of induction of LTP. The enhancement of LTP by NE or ISO occurred with or without picrotoxin in the bath to block GABA-mediated inhibition and thus does not appear to depend on the presence of feedforward or recurrent inhibition.

H. L. Haas   G. Buzsàki (Eds.)
Synaptic Plasticity in the Hippocampus
© Springer-Verlag Berlin Heidelberg 1988

Forskolin (10-50 uM), a diterpene compound that rapidly activates adenylyl cyclase, was also found to enhance LTP, suggesting that an increase in cAMP may be responsible for the effects of NE and ISO on LTP.

We have previously shown that propranolol greatly decreases the probability of induction of LTP at mossy fiber synapses (6). To test whether NE (or ISO) might be acting postsynaptically to increase cAMP

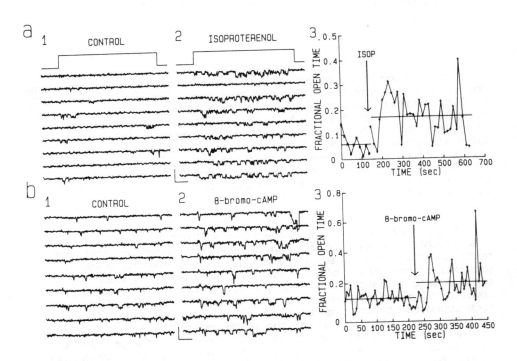

Fig. 1, a. Application of isoproterenol increases the activity of Ca channels in a cell-attached patch from a granule cell. Patch pipettes contained 96 mM BaCl$_2$; 100 uM 3,4-DAP; 1 uM TTX; and 10 mM HEPES; the pH was adjusted to 7.35 with TEA-OH. The exposed cells were bathed in 140 mM K-aspartate; 20 mM dextrose, 1 mM MgCl$_2$; 10 mM EGTA; and 10 mM HEPES. The pH was adjusted to 7.4 with KOH. The K-aspartate saline was used to zero the membrane potential across the whole cell. Voltage jumps were applied to the membrane patch through the patch electrode, and potentials given refer to the patch membrane potential. 1, Consecutive traces of channel activity in control saline in response to step commands from -100 to -10 mV. 2, Channel activity in the same patch 95 s after a 500 ms pressure pulse was applied to a puffer pipette that was located near the cell body and contained bath saline plus 2 uM isoproterenol. 3, Plot of the fraction of time during the command when the current level was more negative than a threshold level (-0.3 pA) before and after application of isoproterenol. The threshold was set at -3 times the standard deviation of the baseline noise calculated from traces in which no channel activity was visible. Each plotted point is the average of three traces, and the horizontal lines indicate the means for all traces before and after drug application. Current traces shown were filtered at 2 kHz (-3 dB, Bessel response) and sampled at 10 kHz. Calibration bar: 2 pA x 10 ms. b. Experiment in which 8-bromo-cAMP was applied in a manner similar to that in a. (From ref. 8)

and enhance LTP, we injected 8-bromo-cAMP into CA3 neurons in slices exposed to propranolol. We found that only cells injected with 8-bromo-cAMP and receiving tetanic stimulation to the mossy fibers displayed LTP. Control cells injected with 5'-AMP or injected with 8-bromo-cAMP but not receiving tetanic stimulation did not exhibit LTP. We also found that during the tetanic stimulation, cells injected with 8-bromo-cAMP had a larger and longer-lasting membrane depolarization than the controls injected with 5'-AMP. These results suggest that the NE (or ISO) enhancement of LTP takes place postsynaptically by increasing the membrane depolarization during tetanic stimulation.

To determine the possible membrane actions of NE that could account for this enhancement of LTP, we made whole-cell and cell-attached patch clamp recordings from hippocampal granule cells. We found that NE, ISO, forskolin, and 8-bromo-cAMP increased whole-cell calcium currents. These agents also produced an increase in the activity of single calcium channels (see Fig. 1). We found no change in single channel conductance, suggesting that the observed increase in whole-cell calcium current is due either to an increase in the channel open time or in the probability of opening of the same or new calcium channels.

It has been shown previously that NE and ISO (and cAMP) decrease the slow afterhyperpolarization following action potentials in hippocampal neurons (10-12). Such a mechanism might lead to greater depolarization and greater calcium influx in the postsynaptic neuron during the LTP induction stimulus if action potentials are triggered postsynaptically during the train. Alternatively, an increase in the activity of calcium channels would also lead to an increase in calcium influx during the train if the membrane potential were sufficiently depolarized to activate the calcium current. With the assumption that a greater calcium influx leads to more LTP, such membrane effects could account for the NE enhancement of LTP.

Supported by NIH grants NS11535, NS15772, HL31164 and AFOSR 85-0178.

REFERENCES

1. Harris, E.W. and Cotman, C.W. Neurosci. Lett. 70: 132-137, 1986.
2. Johnston, D. and Brown, T.H. J. Neurophysiol. 50: 464-486, 1983.
3. Brown, T.H. and Johnston, D. J. Neurophysiol. 50: 487-507, 1983.
4. Barrionuevo, G., Kelso, S.R., Johnston, D. and Brown, T.H. J. Neurophysiol. 55: 540-550, 1986.
5. Griffith, W.H., Brown, T.H. and Johnston, D. J. Neurophysiol. 55: 767-775, 1986.
6. Hopkins, W.F. and Johnston, D. Science 226: 350-352, 1984.
7. Hopkins, W.F. and Johnston, D. (submitted for publication)
8. Gray, R. and Johnston, D. Nature Lond., in press.

9. Gray, R. and Johnston, D. J. Neurophysiol. 54: 134-142, 1985.
10. Madison, D.V. and Nicoll, R.A. Nature Lond. 299: 636-638, 1982.
11. Madison, D.V. and Nicoll, R.A. J. Physiol. Lond. 372: 245-259, 1986.
12. Haas, H.L. and Konnerth, A. Nature Lond. 302: 432-434, 1983.

Potentiation of Synaptic Transmission by Phorbol Esters is Accompanied by a Reduction of Physiological Adenosine Action

P. Schubert

Department of Neuromorphology, Max-Planck Institute for Psychiatry, 8033 Martinsried, Federal Republic of Germany

Removal of the physiological adenosine action by theophylline markedly increased the efficiency of synaptic transmission as determined by measuring the evoked neuronal calcium fluxes in a rat hippocampal slice. The theophylline effect was inhibited by 1 uM phorbol-12,13-dibutyrate and also following generation of LTP.

Phorbol esters were found to enhance transmitter release and to interfere with the stimulation -induced generation of long term potentiation (LTP) (Malenka et al. 1986; 1987). This suggests a similar mode of action involving the activation of protein kinase C (PKC) and underlines the significance of presynaptic mechanisms controlling transmitter release for the maintenance of LTP (Bliss et al. 1986).

In the present paper, we investigated whether an alteration of the modulatory action of adenosine may contribute to changes in the efficiency of synaptic transmission. The latter was determined by measuring the stimulus -induced decreases of the extracellular concentration of calcium ions in the stratum radiatum and in the stratum pyramidale of the rat hippocampal CA1 area. The somatic calcium signal is thought to reflect a voltage -dependent calcium influx into the cell bodies of the target neurons and hence, the amount of post-synaptic activation which is achieved in response to afferent stimulation (see fig. 1).

Even at the low physiological concentration of about 1 uM, adenosine has a strong tonic influence on the efficiency of synaptic transmission. Removal of this

H.L. Haas   G. Buzsàki (Eds.)
Synaptic Plasticity in the Hippocampus
© Springer-Verlag Berlin Heidelberg 1988

adenosine action by adding deaminase or the receptor antagonist theophylline to the superfused medium leads to a marked enhancement of the somatic Ca^{++} signal and may overcome a gradual depression of synaptic transmission exerted in 0.4 mM Ca^{++} medium (fig.1). The effect was considerably increased in the presence of K^+ channel blockers which allowed, even in 0.2 mM Ca^{++} medium, recovery of frequence potentiation (Schubert and Heinemann 1987). This points to a Ca^{++}-dependent presynaptic mechanism and suggests a tonic

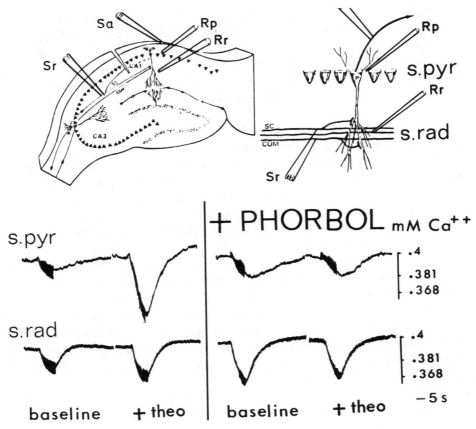

Fig.1 In rat hippocampal slices superfused with a medium containing (in mM): CaCl2 0.4, MgSO4 2.4, KCl 3.3, NaCl 124, NaHCO3 25.7, KH2PO4 1.25, glucose 10, stimulus trains (20 Hz,10 sec) were applied via Sr to the afferent fibers. The evoked decreases in the extracellular Ca^{++} concentration (Ca^{++} signals) were measured with

two ion sensitive/recording electrodes located in the synaptic region (s.rad) and in the soma layer of the CAl pyramidal cells (s.pyr). The Ca^{++} signals generated in the absence and presence of 50 uM theophylline (theo) are shown below, i.e. before (left) and 40 min after addition of 1 uM phorbol-12,13-dibutyrate (right). desensitization of transmitter release to Ca^{++} as a presumable mode of adenosine action.

A change of the sensitivity of the secretory process to Ca^{++} was also described in other systems to result from an activation of PKC (Baker 1984) and may explain the increase of synaptic transmission as observed 20 min after addition of 1 uM phorbol-12,13-dibutyrate to the medium (fig 1). Under these conditions, however, theophylline was no more effective; the Ca^{++} signals were not increased in the presence of this adenosine receptor blocker indicating the absence of adenosine action (fig 1; Schubert 1987, in prep.). The usually observed depression of synaptic transmission is known to be mediated by the Al receptor (Reddington et al. 1982) and it is interesting to note that also another Al receptor -mediated adenosine effect, i.e. the inhibition of cAMP synthesis, has been recently reported to be blocked by phorbol esters (Norstedt and Fredholm 1987). Furthermore, the marked increase of the EPSP amplitude measured in normal medium after addition of theophylline, was reduced by about 60 %, if tested 30 min after the generation of LTP (n=6; p 0.05; see also Lynch and Schubert 1980). These findings support the hypothesis that an LTP -associated activation of PKC leads to a reduction of the Al receptor -mediated depressant effect of adenosine on transmitter release which contributes to the maintenance of LTP.

REFERENCES

Baker PF (1984) Nature 308: 693-698
Bliss TVP, Douglas RM, Errington ML, Lynch MA (1986)
J Physiol London) 377: 391-408
Lynch G, Schubert P (1980) Ann. Rev. Neurosci. 3: 1-22
Malenka RC,Madison D,Nicoll RA (1986) Nature 321:157-177

Malenka RC,Ayoub GS,Nicoll RA (1987) Brain Res 403:198
Norstedt C, Fredholm BF (1987) Naunyn Schmiedeberg's
Arch Pharmacol 335: 136-142
Reddington M, Lee KS, Schubert,P (1982) Neurosci Lett
28:275-279
Schubert P, Heinemann U (1987) Exp Brain Res (submitted)

ACKNOWLEDGEMENT: I thank Prof. G.W. Kreutzberg for
his encouragement of these studies and Maria Koeber for
skillful technical assistance. Supported by SFB 220.

An APV-Resistant Non-associative Form of Long-Term Potentiation in the Rat Hippocampus

J. A. KAUER and R. A. NICOLL

Departments of Pharmacology and Physiology, University of California, San Francisco, CA 94143, USA

Single pyramidal cells of the CA3 region of the hippocampus receive synaptic inputs from two distinct pathways (commissural and mossy fiber) which both exhibit long term potentiation (LTP), but only the commissural LTP is blocked by an NMDA antagonist. Brief tetanization to neighboring synapses fails to potentiate mossy fiber inputs but does potentiate commissural inputs. Thus CA3 pyramidal cells receive synaptic inputs which express fundamentally different forms of synaptic plasticity.

The generation of long term potentiation (LTP) appears to involve two steps: the initiating or trigger event (which may be quite brief) and a long lasting enhancement of the response to synaptic input, which may involve biochemical or structural alterations. Several lines of evidence, primarily from the CA1 region, have suggested that the mechanism underlying the trigger event is a depolarization of the post-synaptic membrane during the synaptic release of glutamate (1-3). Depolarization of the post-synaptic cell appears to relieve a magnesium block of the NMDA subtype of glutamate-activated channel (4). Only when this channel is unblocked can it conduct in response to glutamate released into the synaptic cleft. Application of 2-amino-5-phosphonovaleric acid (APV), a specific blocker of the NMDA receptor subtype, prevents LTP from occurring during high frequency stimulation of an afferent input (5).

Recently field potential recordings from the region of mossy fiber synapses onto CA3 pyramidal cells showed that tetanic stimulation of granule cells in the dentate gyrus produced LTP, even in the presence of APV. In contrast, field recordings in the region of the commissural input to CA3 cells showed the typical reversible blockade of LTP by APV (6). These findings are consistent with anatomical studies suggesting that NMDA receptors are present at very low density in the region of mossy fiber synapses (7).

We now show that two forms of LTP can be observed in pyramidal cells in CA3: the typical associative, APV-sensitive form of LTP described in other areas of the hippocampus, and a novel APV-insensitive form of LTP which is non-associative. Intracellular recordings were made from CA3 pyramidal cells in hippocampal slices while stimulating two separate inputs to these neurons: 1) commissural input with synapses in stratum radiatum, and 2) the mossy fiber terminals synapsing in stratum lucidum. With 50 µM APV in the bath, each input was tetanized twice at 100 Hz for 1 second. The mossy fiber input was strongly potentiated for more than 20 minutes, while the commissural input showed a brief post-tetanic potentiation but returned to baseline levels within a few minutes. Following washout of the APV, the same tetanus to the commissure produced LTP lasting at least 20 minutes.

H.L. Haas   G. Buzsàki (Eds.)
Synaptic Plasticity in the Hippocampus
© Springer-Verlag Berlin Heidelberg 1988

These data show that two different forms of LTP can be observed in pathways synapsing on a single neuron in CA3.

Because of the differential sensitivity of the two forms of LTP to NMDA antagonists, we next compared the ability of these two forms of LTP to exhibit association. Using extracellular recording, we examined the effect of pairing a brief tetanus from one commissural input with a single weak stimulus to a distinct, second commissural input. In agreement with results from CA1 (8) we observed a potentiation of the second input after 8-15 pairings. The brief tetanus presumably depolarizes the post-synaptic cells sufficiently to relieve the Mg^{++} block of the NMDA channels activated by release of transmitter from the weak second input.

In contrast when two mossy fiber inputs were paired in an identical fashion, the single weak input did not change in size or shape, despite the fact that the mossy fibers all terminate in close proximity to one another in stratum lucidum. Following this pairing a homosynaptic tetanus to the weak input produced normal LTP, showing that the synapses were capable of potentiation. The failure to associate could not be attributed to insufficient depolarization, because pairing this same brief mossy fiber tetanus with a commissural EPSP effectively potentiated this commissural input. Thus, while activation of mossy fiber synapses is incapable of modifying neighboring mossy fiber synapses, they can, presumably by providing adequate depolarization, modify more distant commissural synapses.

In summary, these results indicate that CA3 pyramidal cells express two separate forms of LTP, an associative, NMDA-dependent form at the commissural synapses and a non-associative NMDA-independent form from the mossy fiber synapses.

1. Gustafsson, B., Wigström, H., Abraham, W.C. and Huang, Y.-Y. (1987). **Journal of Neuroscience 7,** 774-780.

2. Malinow, R. and Miller, J.P. (1986). **Nature 320,** 529-530.

3. Kelso, S.R., Ganong, A.H. and Brown, T.H. (1986). **Proceedings of the National Academy of Sciences, USA 83,** 5326-5330.

4. Nowak, L., Bregestovski, P., Ascher, P., Herbet, A. and Prochiantz, A. (1984). **Nature 307,** 462-465.

5. Collingridge, G.L., Kehe, S.J. and McLennan, H. (1983). **Journal of Physiology 334,** 33-46.

6. Harris, E.W. and Cotman, C.W. (1986). **Neuroscience Letters 70,** 132-137.

7. Monaghan, D.T. and Cotman, C.W. (1985). **Journal of Neuroscience 5,** 2909-2919.

8. Gustafsson, B. and Wigström, H. (1986). **Journal of Neuroscience 6,** 1575-1582.

GABA Transmission in the Hippocampus: Postsynaptic Regulation

A. Stelzer and R.K.S. Wong

Physiology Institute University of Munich, Munich, Federal Republic of Germany and Department of Neurology, Columbia University, New York, NY 11794, USA

Abstract

The modifiability of the GABA response in the hippocampus has been examined using acutely isolated cells and the slice preparation. The results show that the $GABA_A$-mediated current was regulated by a number of physiologically active substances acting at the intra- or extracellular membrane sites. Mg++ and ATP are essential intracellular components stabilizing the GABA-current. Extracellularly applied excitatory amino acid transmitters and related compounds modulated the GABA-response. Suppression of GABAergic transmission has an important impact in enhancing neuronal excitation following tetanic stimulation in the slice preparation.

It is widely accepted that GABA functions as a neurotransmitter in the mammalian CNS and there is indication that the GABAergic transmission is highly modifiable. Modification can result from alterations in the presynaptic GABA release (1) as well as from changes in the postsynaptic efficacy of the GABA receptor (2). In the present study we examined GABAergic inhibition in the CA1 subfield of the guinea-pig hippocampus focusing on the modifiability at the postsynaptic site. Whole cell voltage-clamp experiments were carried out in acutely isolated pyramidal neurons (3) using low resistance electrodes (2-5 MOhm). All experiments on isolated cells were performed at room temperature. K+ currents were suppressed by external TEA (15mM), CsCl (5mM), 4-AP (5mM) and internally by Tris base (100 mM). GABA (100uM) was applied by short pressure pulses (10-25 msec) of low frequency (0.01 Hz) to prevent cumulative desensitization. In a typical experiment the cell was clamped at -10 mV. We observed that the GABA-induced outward current progressively decreased with time to less than 20 % of the first response in 10 minutes. The rundown of the GABA response was prevented by suitable levels of Mg++ and ATP in the intracellular pipette. A minimum of 3 mM Mg++ in the presence of 2 mM ATP was required for maintaining stable GABA-responses elicited by consecutive pressure pulses. Omission of either Mg++ or ATP resulted in instability of the GABA response.

Under the conditions of stable GABA-currents, we examined the interaction of the GABA-receptor ionophore complex with other transmitter agents. Glutamate (10 uM in the perfusate) reversibly increased the peak amplitude of the GABA current to up to 160% of control. Other structurally related compounds to glutamate such as NMDA and, surprisingly, the NMDA receptor antagonist D-APV produced a similar enhancement of GABA-currents which were also concentration

H.L. Haas   G. Buzsàki (Eds.)
Synaptic Plasticity in the Hippocampus
© Springer-Verlag Berlin Heidelberg 1988

68

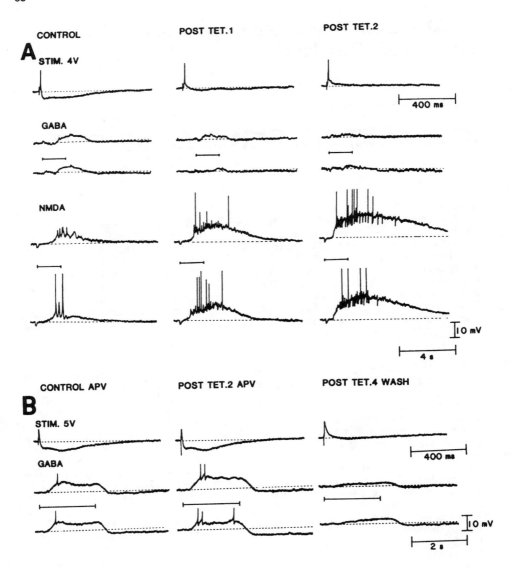

Fig. 1 Effect of tetani on ionophoretically applied GABA and NMDA responses. A,
Progressive fading of the response to applied GABA and the analogous decline of
evoked IPSPs. The NMDA response was greatly enhanced following tetanic stimulation. GABA and NMDA were applied to str. pyramidale through an extracellular 3-
barrelled electrode. B, control GABA response in D-APV, after the second tetanus
in D-APV and after the fourth tetanus following wash. As for inhibitory potentials,
D-APV suppressed the decrease of the response to ionophoretic GABA after repeated tetani. Washout and further tetanization produced a depression of both ortho-
dromically evoked IPSPs and GABA response. Action potential amplitudes in A and
B are attenuated. Horizontal bars under GABA and NMDA responses indicate duration
of drug ejection.

dependent and reversible. Short duration hyperpolarizing voltage pulses applied to estimate the instantaneous leak conductance showed that the GABA-induced conductance was proportionally increased in the presence of the modulating agent. Thus the enhancement of the GABA-current cannot be attributed to changes in the reversal potential.

These results show that the efficacy of the GABA receptors can be modified by physiologically-active substances at both extra- and intracellular membrane sites. The data are particularly interesting in that the modification of GABAergic transmission may contribute to long-term increases of neuronal excitation (Long-term potentiation and epileptiform discharges) following tetanic electrical stimulation.

In another series of experiments (see ref. 4) we have examined the alterations in inhibitory synaptic potentials which accompanied the application of tetanic stimuli to the stratum radiatum fiber input to CA1 pyramidal neurons in the guinea-pig hippocampal slice preparation. Intracellular recordings from CA1 pyramidal neurons revealed a progressive long-lasting reduction of both spontaneous and evoked IPSPs following repetitive tetanization. The reduction of both fast and slow IPSPs was not accompanied by changes in the reversal potential. Further the effects of repeated tetani on IPSPs were compared with the responses of the same cell to ionophoretically applied GABA and NMDA (Fig. 1A).

In these experiments the progressive reduction of IPSPs was matched by a reduction of GABA sensitivity and a large increase in the responsiveness of cells to NMDA. In the presence of D-APV (5-10 uM), tetanization produced no decreases of IPSPs and GABA responses (Fig.1B). Following the washout of D-APV further tetani then produced a fast reduction of both IPSPs and GABA responses.The intrinsic properties of all cells studied remained unchanged. These findings suggest that tetanic stimuli applied to the stratum-radiatum fiber pathway produces a simultaneous reduction in the postsynaptic GABA sensitivity and enhancement of responsiveness to NMDA.

In conclusion these results demonstrate that postsynaptic GABA transmission is highly modifiable by a variety of factors and that modification can occur at both intra- and extracellular membrane sites. Furthermore, decreases in the postsynaptic GABA sensitivity may contribute to a long-term enhancement of neuronal excitation. Although the exact cellular mechanism for suppression of IPSPs following tetanization is not fully clear, it is possible that factors regulating GABA currents in the single cell preparation are effective following the activation of NMDA receptors.

This research was supported by grants from DFG 220 (B2), NIH and the Klingenstein Foundation.

References.

1 Nicoll,R.A., Alger,B.E. and Jahr,C.E., Nature 281,315-317 (1979).

2 Wong,R.K.S. and Watkins,D.J., J. Neurophysiol. 48,938-951 (1982).

3 Kay,A.R. and Wong,R.K.S., J. Neurosc. Methods 16,227-238 (1986).

4 Stelzer,A., Slater,N.T. and ten Bruggencate G., Nature 326, 698-701 (1987).

Glycine Allosterically Regulates an NMDA Receptor Coupled Ion Channel in Rat Hippocampal Membranes

D. W. BONHAUS, B. C. BURGE, J. O. MCNAMARA

Departments of Medicine (Neurology) and Pharmacology, Duke University Medical Center and Epilepsy Research Laboratory, V.A. Medical Center, Durham, NC 27710, USA

N-methyl-D-aspartate (NMDA) receptor mediated neurotransmission plays a crucial role in several forms of neuronal plasticity. In hippocampal slices antagonists of NMDA receptors inhibit long-term potentiation and raise the threshold for evoking seizure-like activity. NMDA receptor agonists likely mediate their effects by activation of a voltage-dependent non-selective cation channel (for review see TINS Vol. 10, 1987).

Glycine, once thought to be an exclusively inhibitory neurotransmitter, was recently found to selectively and dramatically increase the frequency with which NMDA agonists open ion channels in cultured neurons (Johnson and Ascher, 1987). The effect of glycine was specific in that among a variety of amino acids tested only D-serine produced a similar enhancement of NMDA-evoked currents. In contrast to the glycine activated chloride conductance; this response was insensitive to strychnine (1 uM). The mechanism of glycine enhancement of NMDA evoked responses is unknown. One possibility is an allosteric regulation of the NMDA receptor-channel complex itself.

To test this idea we measured the effect of glycine on glutamate dependent binding of the phencyclidine analog $[^3H]$-N-(1-[thienyl-cyclohexyl) piperidine (TCP). Two recent findings indicate that TCP binding can serve as a biochemical marker of NMDA receptor mediated ion channel activation. First, Loo et al. (1986) and others (Fagg, 1987; Foster and Wong, 1987) have shown that NMDA receptor agonists selectively enhance the binding of TCP, a noncompetitive NMDA antagonist, to rat brain membranes. Second, MacDonald et al. (1987) have shown that the noncompetitive NMDA antagonists phencyclidine and ketamine block NMDA evoked currents by a use and voltage dependent mechanism. These findings are consistent with the idea that TCP exerts its noncompetitive block by binding in the lumen of an ion channel which has been opened by the binding of an agonist to the NMDA receptor.

Hippocampal membranes were prepared from adult Sprague-Dawley rats in a 50 mM Tris buffer (pH 7.7) containing 10 mM EDTA. Membranes were extensively washed by repeated homogenization, centrifugation and freeze-thawing. Binding reactions were carried out in a 5 mM Tris buffer (pH 7.7) at 25°C without added EDTA. Specific TCP binding (2.5 nM) was measured as the difference in binding in the presence and absence of 100 uM phencyclidine. Reactions were terminated by vacuum filtration over Whatman GF/B filters. Filters were rinsed with ice-cold Tris buffer and the radioactivity was measured.

Glutamate and NMA (racemic N-methyl-aspartate) but not kainate, increased specific TCP binding in a dose dependent manner; the highest concentrations of glutamate and NMA resulted in a reducton of TCP binding, confirming the findings of Fagg (1987). Addition of 10 uM glycine alone had small and variable effects on specific TCP binding, but dramatically enhanced the poteniating effect of glutamate and NMA (Fig. 1). This effect clearly involved an increase in the efficacy of glutamate and NMA. The potentiation of TCP binding by glycine and glutamate was inhibited by 50 uM D-APV but not by strychnine (1 uM). The effect of glycine was specific in

H. L. Haas   G. Buzsàki (Eds.)
Synaptic Plasticity in the Hippocampus
© Springer-Verlag Berlin Heidelberg 1988

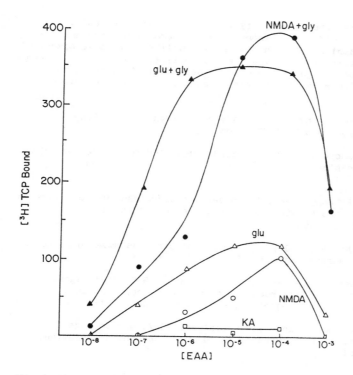

Fig.1. Values are the increase in TCP binding over basal (that seen in the absence of added amino acid) binding (fmoles/mg). Basal TCP binding in the kainate, glutamate and NMA experiments was 88, 130 and 146 fmoles/mg protein respectively. Specific TCP binding was 50% of total binding in the basal condition and was greater than 80% of total binding under conditions of maximal stimulation. Glutamate and NMA but not kainate increased specific TCP binding in a dose dependent manner. Glycine alone had a small effect on TCP binding (15–50 fmoles/mg over basal). Concomitant addition of glycine (10 uM) with either glutamate or NMDA markedly potentiated TCP binding. Comparable results have been obtained in three separate experiments.

that several other amino acids (10 uM; L-cysteine, GABA, glutamine, L-leucine, L-methionine, taurine and L-threonine,) alone had no consistent effect on TCP binding and did not potentiate the action of glutamate on TCP binding. D-serine, 10 uM, did increase glutamate stimulated TCP binding but to a lesser extent than glycine.

These results extend the findings of Johnson and Ascher (1987) and support the hypothesis of a direct physical coupling among an NMDA receptor, a glycine receptor and a cation channel in mammalian hippocampal membranes. The idea that the glycine and NMDA receptors are coupled in a single complex is supported by two findings. First D-APV inhibited the glycine enhancement of TCP binding both in the presence and in the absence of added glutamate. Second, glycine synergistically increased glutamate stimulated TCP binding. This synergistic interaction, rather than a mere additive effect, further supports an allosteric interaction among discrete components of a macromolecular complex, analogous to the GABA-benzodiazepine-barbiturate receptor complex.

These findings raise the possibility that glycine allosterically regulates NMDA receptor mediated responses in the mammalian hippocampus in vivo. Further investiagation of this possibility will require development of a selective antagonist for this strychnine insensitive, NMDA-channel linked, glycine receptor. Glycine regulated glutamate-dependent TCP binding may provide a rapid in vitro assay for screening agonists and antagonists of this receptor.

This work was supported by Veterans Administration Medical Research funds and grants NS 07614 and NS 17771 from the NIH.

Fagg, G.E., 1987, Phyencyclidine and related drugs bind to the activated N-methyl-D-aspartate receptor-channel complex in rat brain membranes, Neurosci. Lett., 76, 221.

Foster, A.C. and E.H.F. Wong, 1987, The novel anticonvulsant MK-801 binds to the activated state of the N-methyl-D-aspartate receptor in rat brain, Br. J. Pharmac. 91, 403.

Johnson, J.W. and P. Ascher, 1987, Glycine potentiates the NMDA response in cultured mouse brain neurons, Nature, 325, 529.

Loo, P., A. Braunwalder, J. Lehmann and M. Williams, 1986, Radioligand binding to central phencyclidine recognition sites is dependent on excitatory amino acid receptor agonists, Eur. J. Pharmacol., 123, 467.

MacDonald, J.f., Z. Miljkovic and P. Pennefather, 1987, Use-dependent block of excitatory amino acid currents in cultured neurons by ketamine, J. Neurophys., 58, 251.

MK-801 Prevents the Induction of Long-Term Potentiation

E. J. COAN, W. SAYWOOD, and G. L. COLLINGRIDGE

Department of Pharmacology, University of Bristol, Bristol, BS8 1TD, United Kingdom

The effects of the pre-incubation of hippocampal slices with MK-801 was examined on synaptic events in the Schaffer collateral-commissural pathway. Treatments which blocked NMDA receptor-mediated synaptic responses also prevented the induction of long term potentiation.

MK-801 ((+)-5-methyl-10,11-dihydro-5H-dibenzo [a,d] cyclo-hepten-5,10-imine maleate) is a potent, non-competitive N-methyl-D-aspartate (NMDA) antagonist (Wong et al, 1986). In this regard it resembles the dissociative anaesthetics phencyclidine and ketamine (Anis et al, 1983) although MK-801 appears to display a marked use-dependence. The purpose of the present investigation was to determine whether MK-801 could, like other NMDA antagonists (see Collingridge and Bliss, 1987), prevent the initiation of long term potentiation (LTP) in the CA1 region of the hippocampus.

Immediately following preparation, transverse rat hippocampal slices were randomly allocated between two petri dishes, where they were pre-incubated in standard (ie 1 mM Mg^{2+}-containing) slice medium, with or without MK-801 for 85-600 min. Slices were then transferred to a recording chamber, which was continuously perfused with standard medium without MK-801, and control and MK-801-treated slices were examined in turn. The Schaffer collateral-commissural pathway was stimulated continuously at a low frequency (0.033 Hz) and field potentials recorded from the CA1 cell body region.

In standard medium there appeared to be no difference in the low frequency synaptic response in control and MK-801-treated slices. With long pre-incubation times some slices developed secondary population spikes indicating deterioration. MK-801-treated slices seemed to deteriorate to a lesser degree.

Since the blocking action of MK-801 is use-dependent experiments were performed to determine the conditions needed for blockade of NMDA receptor-mediated synaptic responses. Following pre-incubation, slices were perfused with Mg^{2+}-free medium for up to 180 min. In controls, low frequency stimulation evoked a large synaptic component that was sensitive to competitive

H. L. Haas   G. Buzsàki (Eds.)
Synaptic Plasticity in the Hippocampus
© Springer-Verlag Berlin Heidelberg 1988

NMDA antagonists (cf Coan and Collingridge, 1985).
Slices that had been pre-incubated with 10 uM MK-801 for
110-270 min displayed little or none of this component
(n=8), indicating that MK-801 pretreatment had caused a
long lasting block of the NMDA receptor system.

To study LTP, slices were stimulated, in standard
medium, at 0.033 Hz for 15-30 min before and for at least
15 min following a period of high frequency stimulation
(100 Hz, 1 s). The criteria for successful LTP was a
stable potentiation of at least 20 % in the population
spike amplitude, 15 min after a high frequency train. In
slices that had been pre-incubated with MK-801 (10 uM)
for 80-440 min it was not possible to elicit LTP (n=14;
Fig. 1A). Indeed, in 7 of these slices, there was a
short-lived depression of the population spike amplitude

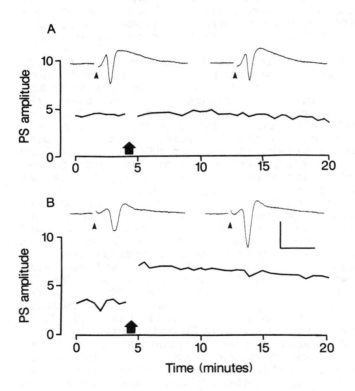

Fig. 1. MK-801 prevents the induction of LTP. A A slice
pre-incubated with 10 uM MK-801 for 200 min. B A slice
from the same rat pre-incubated under control conditions
for 540 min. Each graph plots population spike amplitude
and the arrow indicates time of high frequency
stimulation. Representative records before and 15 min
following high frequency stimulation are shown above.
Calibration bar, 4 mV and 8 ms. Time of stimulation is
shown by arrowheads (stimulus artefacts are blanked).

following high frequency stimulation (Fig. 2). It was possible, however, to induce LTP from 12 of 13 slices which had been prepared from the same rats but incubated without MK-801 (Fig. 1B). The mean (+ 1 S.E.) potentiation of controls 15 min following high frequency stimulation was 61 + 12 %.

These data demonstrate that MK-801 can, like competitive NMDA antagonists (Collingridge et al, 1983) and dissociative anaesthetics (Stringer and Guyenet, 1983), block the induction of LTP in the CA1 region of the hippocampus. It has been reported, however, that MK-801 does not block the production of LTP in the perforant path input to the dentate gyrus in vivo (Halliwell and Morris, 1987). This may have been due to problems with achieving blockade with MK-801 of the dentate NMDA receptor system since competitive NMDA antagonists prevent the induction of LTP in both medial and lateral components of this pathway (see Collingridge and Bliss, 1987).

In conclusion these data support the idea that NMDA receptors are involved in the induction of LTP and suggest that MK-801 may impair some cognitive functions.

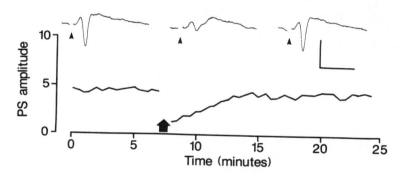

Fig. 2. MK-801 can cause short-term depression following high frequency stimulation. This slice had been pre-incubated with 10 uM MK-801 for 230 min. Records show the response before, 1 min and 15 min following high frequency stimulation. (cf Fig. 1. for details).

References

Anis NA, Berry SC, Burton NR, Lodge D (1983) The dissociative anaesthetics, ketamine and phencyclidine, selectively reduce excitation of central mammalian neurones by N-methyl-D-aspartate. Br J Pharmac 79: 565-575

Coan EJ, Collingridge GL (1985) Magnesium ions block an N-methyl-D-aspartate receptor-mediated component of synaptic transmission in rat hippocampus. Neurosci Lett 53: 21-26

Collingridge GL, Bliss TVP (1987) NMDA receptors- their role in long-term potentiation. TINS 10: 288-293

Collingridge GL, Kehl SJ, McLennan H (1983) Excitatory amino acids in synaptic transmission in the Schaffer collateral-commissural pathway of the rat hippocampus. J Physiol (Lond) 334: 33-46

Halliwell RF, Morris RGM (1987) Systemic doses of MK-801 fail to block long-term potentiation in vivo or impair spatial memory in the rat. Neurosci Lett Suppl 29: S99

Stringer JL, Guyenet PG (1983) Elimination of long-term potentiation in the hippocampus by phencyclidine and ketamine. Brain Res 258: 159-164

Wong EHF, Kemp JA, Priestley T, Knight AR, Woodruff GN, Iversen LL (1986) The anticonvulsant MK-801 is a potent N-methyl-D-aspartate antagonist. Proc Natl Acad Sci USA 83: 7104-7108

Long-Term Potentiation in Slices from Human Hippocampus

H. L. HAAS, R. W. GREENE, B. HEIMRICH, and X. XIE

Neurochirurgische Universitätsklinik 8091 Zürich, Switzerland and Department of Physiology, University of Mainz, 6500 Mainz, Federal Republic of Germany

Abstract

Long-term potentiation (LTP) has been observed in slices from human hippocampi removed for intractable epilepsy using extra- and intracellular recording in vitro. Furthermore the effects of several neuroactive substances with possible relevance for synaptic plasticity was investigated. Human hippocampal neurones in vitro display properties very similar to the respective rodent cells.

Introduction and methods

Experiments on slices from human neocortex have previously been described but, to our knowledge, this ist the first report on intracellular recordings from the human hippocampus. Slices were prepared from hippocampi immediately after removal from patients suffering from temporal lobe epilepsy (en bloc unilateral hippocampamygdalectomy, M.G. Yasargil) and investigated in an in vitro perfusion chamber for periods upto 15 hours. Slices were cut with a razor blade using a perspex guide, transferred to a large perfusion chamber (Haas et al., 1979) and investigated with extra- and intracellular recording (current- and voltage clamp).

Results

Field potentials, in particular the population spikes recorded in the cell layers following electrical stimulation of afferent fibers to the CA 1 and dentate regions were similar to those described in hippocampal slices of rodents. They were, however, comparatively small (0.5-5 mV). Dendritic potentials were negative but the typical shape was not seen. Although these hippocampi had generated epileptic discharges in vivo, spontaneous epileptiform potentials were never observed in vitro.

Tetanization (100-400 Hz for 40 to 1000 ms) was followed by a comparatively small posttetanic potentiation and occasionally by LTP of the synaptically evoked population spikes and the intracellularly registered epsp-ipsp sequence. LTP was observed in 5 slices from 2 patients for at least 20 min after tetanisation (100-400 Hz for 40-1000 ms) (Figs. 1 and 2). In a much larger number of experiments however, no potentiation or a long lasting depression was found. In slices from 12 further patients where only fibre potentials could be

H. L. Haas   G. Buzsàki (Eds.)
Synaptic Plasticity in the Hippocampus
© Springer-Verlag Berlin Heidelberg 1988

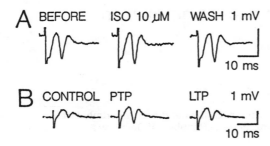

A BEFORE   ISO 10 μM   WASH 1 mV

                                    10 ms

B CONTROL PTP   LTP   1 mV

                                    10 ms

Fig. 1. Population spikes recorded from the dentate cell layers of human hippo-
campal slices. All potentials are averages of 8 sweeps. A: Perfusion with 10 uM
isoproterenol (beta-agonist) caused a small and partially permanent increase in
the population spikes (WASH 20 min after withdrawal of isoproterenol). B: Post-
tetanic potentiation (PTP) (average between 30 s and 2 min after tetanus) and
long-term potentiation (LTP, 20 min after tetanus).

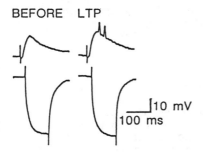

BEFORE LTP

                        ]10 mV
            100 ms

Fig. 2. Long-term potentiation recorded from a CA1 pyramidal cell in a human
hippocampal slice. All traces are averages from 8 sweeps. Upper traces illustra-
te the depolarizing epsp-ipsp sequence recorded with a KCl filled electrode.

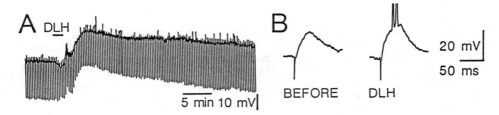

A DLH   B

                    5 min 10 mV| 20 mV|
                                              50 mV|
                                  BEFORE   DLH

Fig. 3. The effects of D,L-homocysteic acid (DLH) on CA1 cells in human hippo-
campal slices. Perfusion was for 1 min with 1 mM DLH (bolus application). A: A
long lasting depolarisation. Resting potential was ca. 70 mV, downward excur-
sions are from -0.5 nA current injections. B: In a different cell the membrane
potential during the response to DLH was manually clamped tò the original res- ·
ting potential (ca. 70 mV). The synaptic potential(depolarizing epsp-ipsp se-
quence recorded with KCl filled electrode) was enhanced during DLH action. This
effect may be due to activation of NMDA receptors by DLH, in particular the grea-
ter steepness of the initial component, but could also reflect a facilitated dis-
charge of inhibitory interneurones.

recorded (Haas et al., 1983) tetanisation did not affect these fibre spikes for periods longer than a few minutes.

A number of neuroactive substances with possible relevance to synaptic plasticity were added to the perfusion fluid: D,L-homocysteic acid (1mM bolus application) depolarized 2 cells by 15 mV and increased the synaptic potential (Fig. 3). Carbachol (1uM) depolarized one cell by 3 mV, decreased the conductance by 12.5 %, blocked the accommodation of firing during depolarizing current injection, and reduced the synaptic potential. Serotonin (10 uM) hyperpolarized one cell by 6 mV and increased the membrane conductance by 50%. During washout, an opposite effect was observed: depolarization and a reduction in accommodation of firing. Baclofen (5uM) hyperpolarized one cell by 6 mV and increased conductance by 25% (measured at the resting voltage, -69 mV). Adenosine (10-100 uM) hyperpolarized 3 cells by 6,7,10 mV and caused an outward current of 150 pA (1 cell, 10 uM). Long lasting afterhyperpolarizations, accommodation of firing and an outward tail current after depolarizing voltage jumps were enhanced. Histamine (5 uM) blocked the accommodation of firing in one cell. Isoproterenol caused a small permanent increase in population spikes in two experiments on the dentate region (Fig. 1).

Discussion

The results demonstrate a remarkable consistency in basic cell functions between rodents and man in spite of the greater complexity of human hippocampal circuitry and thus emphasize the validity of animal models in studying cellular neurophysiology.
Appendix: We have previously described LTP of the epsp-ipsp sequence as shown in fig. 2. with intracellular recording using a KCl filled electrode in rat slices (Haas and Rose, 1982; Haas and Greene, 1985; Haas, 1986). In these papers we have also reported the failure of evoking LTP in CA 1 cells filled with caesium chloride. However, Griffith et al. (1986) were able to demonstrate LTP by recording synaptic currents in CA 3 with such electrodes. A possible explanation of this discrepancy is the fact that in our current clamp experiments Ca-spikes were often fired by the paired synaptic potentials during the control period before the tetanus. These may have saturated the LTP inducing mechanism before tetanization. There was indeed for some time after impalement of a cell a continuous increase of the synaptic potential – an effect we have originally attributed to the increasing concentration of caesium in the cell.

References

Griffith, W.H., Brown, T.H. & Johnston, D. (1986) Voltage-clamp analysis of synaptic inhibition during long-term potentiation in hippocampus. J. Neurophysiol. 55, 767-775.
Haas, H.L. (1986) Long-term potentiation and intrinsic disinhibition. In: Learning and Memory: Mechanisms of information storage in the nervous system. Ed. H. Matthies, Advances in the Biosciences Vol. 59, 41-49, Pergamon, Oxford.
H.L. Haas and R.W. Greene (1985) Long-term potentiation and 4-aminopyridine. Cell.Mol.Neurobiol. 5, 297-301.

Haas, H.L. & Rose, G. (1982). Long-term potentiation of excitatory synaptic transmission in the rat hippocampus: the role of inhibitory processes. J. Physiol. 329, 541-552.

Haas, H.L. & Rose, G. (1984). The role of inhibitory mechanisms in hippocampal long term potentiation. Neurosci. Lett. 47, 301-306.

Haas, H.L., Schärer, B. & Vosmansky, M. (1979). A simple perfusion chamber for the study of nervous tissue slices in vitro. J. of Neuroscience Meth. 1, 323-325.

Haas, H.L., Wieser, H.G. and Yasargil, M.G. (1983). 4-Aminopyridine and fiber potentials in rat and human hippocampal slices. Experientia 39, 114-115.

Decrease of GABA During Long-Term Potentiation in the CA1 Region of Rat Hippocampal Slices: Immunohistochemical and Biochemical Analysis

Y. Horikawa, H. Okamura[1], I. Hirotsu, T. Ishihara, T. Hashimoto[2], K. Kuriyama[2], H. Kimura[3], and Y. Ibata[1]

Suntory Institute for Biomedical Research, Laboratory for Experimental Pharmacology, Shimamotocho, Osaka 618; Kyoto Pref. University Medical, Departments of [1]Anatomy and [2]Pharmacology, Kyoto 602; Shiga University Medical Sciences, [3]Department of Anatomy, Otsu, Japan

Abstract

To elucidate the participation of hippocampal interneurons on the occurrence of long-term potentiation (LTP), the functional change in GABA-ergic neurons during LTP was investigated in hippocampal slices immunocytochemically using anti-GABA serum, as well as neurochemically by HPLC procedures. Pyramidal GABA-like immunoreactive neurons had a decreased immunoreactivity in neuronal perikarya and terminal varicosities surrounding pyramidal cells of CA1 in LTP slices compared with those in controls. These changes were not observed in the other regions of CA1 or during short-term potentiation (STP). GABA concentration in CA1-CA3 regions displayed a significant reduction (28%) during LTP ($P < 0.05$). These results suggested that the function of GABA-ergic interneurons in str. pyramidale may be altered during LTP.

Introduction

Long-term potentiation (LTP) in the hippocampus is a long lasting enhancement of the post synaptic evoked response following high frequency repetitive stimulation (tetanus) of afferents, which is considered to be a model of the neuronal plasticity. The involvement of interneurons in the LTP phenomenon is unclear [2,5]. The physiologically defined inhibitory interneurons are most often associated with the immunocytochemically identified GABA-like immunoreactive [-LI] or GAD-LI neurons. We investigated the morphological changes in GABA-LI neurons of CA1 during LTP by electrophysiology combined with immunocytochemistry using anti-GABA serum.

Electrophysiological conditions

Hippocampal slices (400 μm thickness) from Fischer rats (4 W) were prepared in the usual way [11]. Electrical stimuli were delivered to the Schaffer collaterals of the CA3/CA2 junction and recordings were obtained extracellulary from CA1 pyramidal cell layers. Electrophysiological conditions were as follows : Group 1 ; for control, slices were given only test stimuli (0.2 Hz, 50 μsec, 0.7-0.9 mA) for 60min. Group 2 ; for LTP, slices were given the same treatment as group1 except for a single tetanus (200 Hz, 1 sec). Group 3 ; for STP, slices were taken out immediately after tetanus. LTP was about 200 % of the control level 60 min after the tetanus.

Immunocytochemical procedures applied to hippocampal slices

After the electrophysiological experiments, the slices were immersed in a fixative containing 2 % paraformaldehyde, 0.35 % glutaraldehyde, and 0.2 % picric acid in 0.1 M phosphate-buffer (pH 7.4) for 2 hr. They were then placed in the fixative without glutaraldehyde for 12 hr at 4 °C.

H.L. Haas G. Buzsàki (Eds.)
Synaptic Plasticity in the Hippocampus
© Springer-Verlag Berlin Heidelberg 1988

Sections (40 μm) were made from the slices by a microslicer. The sections were processed for ABC immunocytochemistry as modified for free-floating sections, with affinity purified anti-GABA serum diluted 1/5000. The preparation of the antibody and its specificty have been described elsewhere [9]. Positive GABA-LI staining was completely abolished by preabsorption of the antiserum with GABA (200-1000nmole/ml). For more precise observations of GABA-LI varicosities, some of these sections were embedded in EPON mixture and 1 μm thick sections were also prepared.

Distribution of GABA-LI neurons in control slices (group 1)
The immunocytochemical distribution of GABA-LI neurons in control slices was in agreement with the reports using antiserum of GAD [10] or GABA [9]. Moreover the immunocytochemical distribution pattern was not affected by test stimuli applied for 60 min at intervals of 5 min. GABA-LI neurons were distributed in all layers of CA1 except alveus, and were divided into three main classes : the superficial part of str. oriens, str. pyramidale, and the deep part of str. radiatum/str. lacunosum-moleculare. GABA-LI fibers and terminals were abundantly distributed in all layers of CA1.

Influence of LTP on GABA-LI neurons
In the LTP group, the number and staining intensity of GABA-LI perikarya was reduced particularly in str. pyramidale, compared with the control group in 40 μm sections (Fig.1 a,b). In 1 μm EPON-embedded sections, the number of GABA-LI terminal varicosities was reduced around the pyramidal cells (Fig.1 c,d). GABA-LI neurons located in the other layers, however, did not change immunoreactivity. No pathological changes in the structure of cells were observed in HE stained sections of LTP. In the STP group, the immunoreactivity for anti-GABA serum was the same as in the control group, and did not show the reduction of GABA-LI in str. pyramidale.
Thus we speculate this phenomenon is LTP-associated.

Chemical determination of GABA during LTP
We performed a chemical assay for GABA during LTP in comparison with control slices which comfirmed the above mentioned immunocytochemical changes. After completion of the electrophysiological experiments on slices containing only CA1-CA3, they were homogenized by sonication and were then centrifuged at 3000 rpm for 10 min. The supernatant thus obtained was directly applied to high-performance liquid chromatography (HPLC) with fluorometric detection. The content of GABA was significantly reduced in the LTP group (control : 9.47 ± 0.93, LTP : 6.96 ± 0.57, Mean $\pm$ S.E., nmole/mg protein, $P < 0.05$), whereas there was no significant change in glutamic acid, aspartic acid and glycine. Thus we conclude that the GABA content in interneurons is indeed diminished during LTP.

GABA-ergic neuron and LTP
The LTP-associated decrease of GABA-LI varicosities on pyramidal cell surfaces as shown in the present study may indicate that recurrent inhibition is altered during LTP. It has been reported that the EPSP-population spike curve shifts to the left in the potentiated condition, i.e. for a given EPSP there are larger population spikes [1,4]. Although our immunocytochemical result does not show release of GABA directly, a decrease of recurrent inhibition on pyramidal cell surfaces may contribute to a shift of the E-S amplitude curve in LTP. A decrease in the release of GABA in vivo during LTP was reported by Bliss

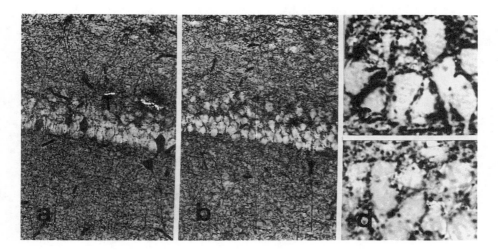

Fig.1 GABA-LI staining of CA1 in control (a,c) and in LTP (b,d).
Note GABA-LI perikarya (b) and terminal varicosities surrounding
pyramidal cells (c) are reduced during LTP. Thickness of sections ;
(a,b) 40 μm , (c,d) 1 μm. (a,b X 140,   c,d X 270)

et al. [3]. Electron microscopic studies found morphological changes of
synapses on interneuron dendrites during LTP [6,8]. Our
immunocytochemical result revealed a decrease of GABA content in
interneurons during LTP.

References

 1 Abraham, W. C., Bliss, T. V. P. and Goddard, G. V., J. Physiol.,
   363, 335-349 (1985)
 2 Andersen, P. and Hvalby, ø., In R. L. Isaacson and K. H. Pribram.
   (Eds.), The Hippocampus 3, New York, Plenum Press., 169-186 (1986)
 3 Bliss, T. V. P., Douglas, R. M., Errington, M. L. and Lynch, M. A.,
   J. Physiol., 377, 391-408 (1986)
 4 Bliss, T. V. P. and Lomo, T., J. Physiol., 232, 331-356 (1973)
 5 Buzsáki, G. and Eidelberg, E., J. Neurophysiol., 48, 597-607 (1982)
 6 Chang, F. -L. F. and Greenough, W. T., Brain Res., 309, 35-46 (1984)
 7 Gamrani, H., Onteniente, B., Seguela, P., Geffard, M. and Calas,
   A., Brain Res., 364, 30-38 (1986)
 8 Lee, K. S., Schottler, F., Oliver, M. and Lynch, G., J. Neurophysiol.,
   44, 247-258 (1980)
 9 Onteniente, B., Tago, H., Kimura, H. and Maeda, T., J. Comp. Neurol.,
   248, 422-430 (1986)
10 Ribak, C. E., Vaughn, J. E. and Saito, K., Brain Res., 140, 315-332
   (1978)
11 Yamamoto, C. and Chujo, T., Exp. Neurol., 58, 242-250 (1978)

What Does Long-Term
Potentiation Model?

Synaptic Organization of Identified Neurons in the Hippocampus

M. FROTSCHER

Institute of Anatomy, Johann-Wolfgang-Goethe-Universität, Theodor-Stern-Kai 7,
6000 Frankfurt am Main 70, Federal Republic of Germany

Abstract

Pyramidal neurons of the hippocampus proper and granule cells of the fascia dentata form the majority of hippocampal neurons and are thus regarded as the target structures of hippocampal afferents. The present study shows, by employing anterograde axonal degeneration, combined Golgi electron microscopy (EM), and immunocytochemical methods, that hippocampal afferents (commissural fibers, septohippocampal cholinergic afferents) and intrahippocampal fiber systems (GABAergic terminals, mossy fibers) also terminate on inhibitory GABAergic nonpyramidal neurons. Functional implications of these connections, such as feed-forward inhibition and disinhibition of pyramidal neurons and granule cells, are considered.

Hippocampal afferents are known to terminate in a laminated fashion in the different layers of the hippocampus and fascia dentata. Pyramidal neurons and dentate granule cells, which are the prevailing cell types of the hippocampus, extend their dendrites to all these layers and are therefore regarded as the targets of hippocampal afferents. However, in addition to these main types of hippocampal neuron, there is a variety of so-called nonpyramidal cells in the hippocampus which are distributed over all layers. Most of them are GABAergic but a few nonpyramidal neurons have been found which react with antibodies against the acetylcholine-synthesizing enzyme choline acetyltransferase (ChAT) (Frotscher et al. 1986). Neuroactive peptides such as cholecystokinin (CCK), vasoactive intestinal polypeptide (VIP), and somotostatin are co-localized with GABA in nonpyramidal neurons (Somogyi et al. 1984; Kosaka et al. 1985). Many GABAergic neurons most likely represent the basket cells known to form a dense pericellular network around the cell bodies of pyramidal neurons and granule cells (Cajal 1911; Lorente de Nó 1934). In fact, immunocytochemical studies have shown that GABAergic boutons form numerous symmetric synaptic contacts on cell bodies, proximal dendrites and axon initial segments of pyramidal neurons and granule cells (e.g. Somogyi et al. 1983; Kosaka et al. 1984).

H.L. Haas   G. Buzsàki (Eds.)
Synaptic Plasticity in the Hippocampus
© Springer-Verlag Berlin Heidelberg 1988

Since GABA is the inhibitory transmitter of the hippocampus these neurons may very effectively control the discharge of hippocampal principal cells. They are known to be activated by recurrent collaterals of pyramidal cell axons.

Golgi preparations demonstrate that dendrites of nonpyramidal neurons often traverse all hippocampal layers, as do dendrites of pyramidal neurons. Hence, the dendrites of nonpyramidal neurons might also be contacted by the various hippocampal afferents terminating in these layers. These suggestions are supported by Golgi/EM studies which revealed numerous synaptic contacts on the varicose dendrites of nonpyramidal cells. In CA3 large mossy fiber boutons were found which established synaptic contacts with both large spines (excrescences) of pyramidal neurons and smooth dendrites of nonpyramidal cells. This latter connection provides a morphological basis for <u>feed-forward inhibition</u> in this region: The excitatory mossy fibers, most likely using glutamate as transmitter, activate inhibitory nonpyramidal neurons which in turn inhibit the pyramidal cells. Contacts with both pyramidal and nonpyramidal neurons have similarly been observed in case of commissural afferents from the contralateral hippocampus. In these studies anterograde axonal degeneration was used to label commissural fibers and the Golgi/EM procedure or GAD immunocytochemistry to identify postsynaptic GABAergic nonpyramidal cells. By employing electron microscopic double immunostaining, we were recently able to demonstrate that cholinergic septohippocampal afferents terminate on GABAergic nonpyramidal neurons, in addition to their contacts on pyramidal and granule cells. Finally, electron microscopy of GAD-immunostained sections revealed symmetric synaptic contacts between GABAergic terminals and GABAergic cell bodies. Such connection may indicate inhibition of inhibitory neurons eventually leading to <u>disinhibition</u> of pyramidal neurons and granule cells.

In conclusion, all hippocampal afferents examined so far have been found to synapse on both principal and nonpyramidal neurons. These results have to be taken into consideration in electrophysiological studies, for instance in studies on synaptic plasticity in the hippocampus.

<u>Acknowledgements</u>

Parts of these studies were performed in close collaboration with Drs. C. Leranth (Section of Neuroanatomy, Yale Univ. School of Med., New Haven), U. Misgeld (Max-Planck-Institut für Psychiatrie, München), and J. Zimmer (Institute of Anatomy B, University of Aarhus). The technical assistance of E. Thielen and E. Schreiber is gratefully acknowledged. This work was supported by the Deutsche Forschungsgemeinschaft: SFB 45, Fr 620/1-3, Fr 620/2-2.

References

Cajal, S.R.y: Histologie du système nerveux de l' homme et des vertébrés. Vol II (1911) A. Maloine, Paris.

Frotscher,M., M.Schlander and C.Leranth: Cell Tissue Res. 246 (1986) 293-301.

Kosaka,T., K.Hama and J.-Y.Wu: Brain Res. 293 (1984) 353 - 359.

Kosaka,T., K.Kosaka, K.Tateishi, Y.Hamaoka, N.Yanaihara, J.Y.Wu and K.Hama: J. Comp. Neurol. 239 (1985) 420-430.

Lorente de Nó,R.: J. Psychol. Neurol. 46 (1934) 113-177.

Somogyi,P., A.J.Hodgson, A.D.Smith, M.G.Nunzi, A.Gorio and J.Y.Wu: J. Neurosci. 4 (1984) 2590-2603.

Somogyi,P., A.D.Smith, M.G.Nunzi, A.Gorio, H.Takagi and J.Y.Wu: J. Neurosci. 3 (1983) 1450-1468.

Hippocampal Sharp Waves: A Physiological Correlate of LTP?

G. Buzsàki and H. L. Haas

Department of Physiology, Medical School, Pécs, Hungary and Department of Physiology, University of Mainz, 6500 Mainz, Federal Republic of Germany

The irregularly occurring large amplitude hippocampal sharp waves (SPWs) are correlated with synchronous population bursts of CA1-CA3 and subicular pyramidal cells, dentate granule cells and interneurons in all hippocampal fields. We suggest that the SPW-associated neuronal burst is the best candidate for a physiological basis of long-term potentiation (LTP).

During consummatory behaviors, immobility, and slow wave sleep, irregular SPWs at 0.01 to 2 Hz may be recorded from all hippocampal fields (Buzsàki 1986; Fig. 1). They can occur isolated or in groups of several successive waves (40-150 msec in duration, 1 to 3.5 mV). The interwave interval within the SPW-burst varies from 50 to 200 msec. Concurrent with the SPWs a large number of pyramidal cells in all hippocampal fields fire in bursts of 2 to 7 action potentials. The synchronous discharge of a large group of pyramidal cells may form a series of "mini" population spikes at 50-200/sec in the pyramidal layer (Fig. 1f). Interneurons and granule cells also increase their discharge rates during the population burst. SPWs occur synchronously in both hippocampi, thus pyramidal cells may be excited via the associational and commissural fibers in a cooperative manner.

Synchronous activation of several input fibers is required to produce LTP. We suggest that the optimal stimulation parameters for LTP to produce long-term neuronal changes, as observed empirically, are similar to the SPW-associated population bursts. LTP is most reliably elicited by short trains of 50 to 400 Hz stimuli (Douglas and Goddard 1975). This frequency is similar to the repetition frequency of "mini" population spikes during the SPW. The high frequency bursts are most effective if repeated by 100-200 msec intervals (Larson and Lynch 1986, Sastry et al. 1986), which is similar to intervals between the SPWs during a SPW burst.

H. L. Haas   G. Buzsàki (Eds.)
Synaptic Plasticity in the Hippocampus
© Springer-Verlag Berlin Heidelberg 1988

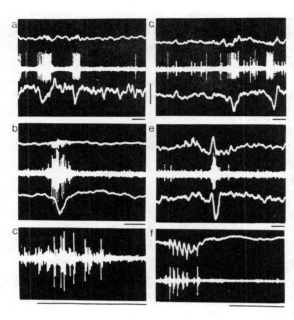

FIG. 1. Correlation between field SPWs and neuronal activity in awake rats. a-d. same rat. a. interneuron in CA1 pyramidal layer. b. and c. multiunit bursts in CA1 pyramidal layer. d. granule cell. e. SPW-associated burst in hilus. f. "mini" population spikes on the peak of SPW recorded just below CA1 pyramdial layer. Upper records: local EEG. Lower records: EEG from a fixed electrode in str. radiatum of CA1. 1 mV, 0.2 sec.

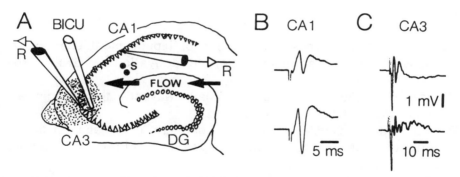

FIG. 2. A diagram of a hippocampal slice showing the location of the stimulating (S), the recording (R) electrodes, and the bicuculline/methylene blue-containing pipette (BICU). The hatched area shows the typical extent of bicuculline/methylene blue diffusion. B. Averages of 8 evoked responses in CA1 pyramidal layer before (above) and 20 min after (below) bicuculline application to the CA3 region. Potentiation was observed up to 90 min. C. Antidromic responses in CA3 before (above) and during (below) bicuculine application near the recording electrode in CA3 pyramidal layer.

Artificially induced population bursts in CA3 region, triggered by single pulse stimulation in the presence of bicuculline, produced LTP in the target CA1 region (Fig. 2). In these experiments bicuculline was applied locally to the CA3 region and a series of small population spikes, similar to the "mini" population spikes during the SPW, was induced by antidromic single pulses. The potentiation outlasted the local effects of bicuculline on the CA3 cells and thus represents a true long-term synaptic change. Conversely, high frequency stimulation of the Schaffer collaterals in vivo increased the amplitude and frequency of the spontaneous SPWs for several hours (Buzsáki 1984).

Our results provide new insights into the possible physiological mechanisms which might be responsible for LTP under natural conditions. They suggest that the neuronal mechanisms underlying hippocampal SPWs meet the criteria of LTP-inducing conditions. Our data also provides a basis to argue that LTP may be a mechanism for long-term pathological changes (e.g., epilepsy) following transient excitability changes.

References:

Buzsáki G (1984) Long-term changes of hippocampal sharp-waves following high frequency afferent activation. Brain Res. 300:179-182.
Buzsáki G (1986) Hippocampal sharp waves: their origin and significance. Brain Res. 398:242-252.
Douglas RM and Goddard G (1975) Long-term potentiation of the perforant path granule cell synapse in the rat hippocampus. Brain Res. 86:205-215.
Larson J and Lynch G (1986) Induction of synaptic potentiation in hippocampus by patterned stimulation involves two events. Science 232:985-988.
Sastry BR, Goh JW and Auyeung A (1986) Associative induction of posttetanic and long-term potentiation in CA1 neurons of rat hippocampus. Science 232:988-990.

Characteristics of Associative Potentiation/Depression

W. B. LEVY and N. L. DESMOND

Department of Neurological Surgery, University of Virginia School of Medicine,
Charlottesville, VA 22903, USA

Studies of the monosynaptic, bilateral entorhinal cortex (EC) – dentate gyrus (DG) responses are being used to choose among the numerous synaptic modification rules suggested in neurodynamic theories of concept formation and pattern recognition. The EC–DG system has many advantages, including (a) numerous available controls [1], (b) the wealth of anatomical and physiological knowledge about the system [2], and (c) the use of bilaterally placed, widely separated stimulating electrodes [1]. In addition, there is the fact that the requisite stimulation intensity and response amplitude of the contralateral EC–DG pEPSP have no lower limits that restrict the phenomenology of associative potentiation/depression. That is, so long as a contralateral response is measurably above noise levels and a powerful converging ipsilateral response is available, then all of our reported results for long-term potentiation and depression hold for the weak contralateral response. These results encourage an extrapolation in which only a single EC–DG fiber is activated. This extrapolation, the specificity and individuality of contralateral modifiability [1,3,4,5], the synaptic modification correlates of LTP revealed by electron microscopy [6,7], and the existence of a suitable molecular mechanism to explain associative potentiation (i.e. the voltage–controlled NMDA receptor [8]), further encourage us to study synaptic modification in the EC–DG system in order to properly formalize the rule of associative modification.

To conform with our electrophysiological data, the formalized rule needs at least three characteristics. This rule must treat long-term potentiation and depression equivalently [3,4]. It must limit potentiation or depression to some asymptotic value under repetitive stimulation conditions [4,5]. Finally, the rule must show threshold properties [9,10].

As a starting point, we consider the synaptic strength of a synapse made by cell i with cell j at time t, i.e. $W_{ij}(t)$, with the units of this quantity left unspecified. A synaptic modification updating rule is just like a synaptic modification experiment

$$W_{ij}(t+1) = W_{ij}(t) + \Delta W_{ij}(t).$$

That is, the synaptic strength at time (t+1) is the synaptic strength at time (t) plus the change that occurs over the interval between (t) and (t+1). The heart of the modification rule is the form of $\Delta W_{ij}(t)$. For notational simplicity, we now drop reference to time while remembering that the synaptic modification rule must conform to the observed temporal dependencies of associative potentiation/depression

H.L. Haas   G. Buzsàki (Eds.)
Synaptic Plasticity in the Hippocampus
© Springer-Verlag Berlin Heidelberg 1988

[11]. The simplest form that fits the above results is

$$\Delta W_{ij} = \varepsilon \cdot f(\text{postsynaptic excitation}_j) \cdot (X_i - W_{ij} \cdot C).$$

Here X_i is the frequency of the test afferent. ε represents a nonspecific term ranging in value from 0 to 1. $f(\ )$ is a sigmoid (or even an off-on step) function operating on the net postsynaptic excitation of cell j, with values from 0 to 1 (or 0 or 1). C is a constant expressed in units which ensure that the terms of the subtraction are in the same units.

Recent experiments with repetitive potentiation and then depression of the same responses indicate that modifiability decreases as a function of the amount of previous modification in a way not predicted by the usual synaptic modification equation. Incorporating this result with a threshold, on-off type postsynaptic permissive event led to a modification rule suitable for Bayesian learning.

$$\Delta W_{ij} = \frac{f_j(X,W) \cdot (X_i - W_{ij} \, C)}{d + \sum\limits_{t} f_j(X,W)}$$

Here $f_j(\ )$ is the same postsynaptic term taking on values 0 or 1, d is a positive constant, and the summation of the denominator is over all past time. When a suitable starting point is selected for time zero so that

$$W_{ij}(0) = \frac{a}{d} \quad \text{with } 0 < \frac{a}{d} < 1,$$

then at any later time (T)

$$W_{ij}(T) = \frac{a + \sum\limits_{t=0}^{T} f_j(X,W) X_i(t)}{d + \sum\limits_{t=0}^{T} f_j(X,W)}.$$

This equation is just the Bayesian's way of estimating the conditional probability of X_i given $f_j(\ )$.

Supported in part by NIH NS15488 and NIMH RSDA MH00622 to WBL.

References

[1] Levy, W. B & Desmond, N. L (1985) In: Electrical Activity of the Archicortex. (G. Buzsaki & C. H. Vanderwolf, Eds.), Budapest: Akademiai Kiado, pp. 359-373.
[2] Andersen, P., Holmqvist, B., & Voorhoeve, P. E. (1966) Acta Physiol. Scand. 66:448-460.
[3] Burger, B. S. & Levy, W. B (1983) Soc. Neurosci. Abstr. 9:1221.
[4] Burger, B., Dickstein, R. & Levy, W. B (1984) Soc. Neurosci. Abstr. 10:77.

[5] Lopez, H., Burger, B. & Levy, W. B (1985) Soc. Neurosci. Abstr. 11:930.

[6] Desmond, N. L & Levy, W. B (1983) Brain Res. 265:21-30.

[7] Desmond, N. L & Levy, W. B (1987) In: Long-Term Potentiation: From Biophysics to Behavior. (P. A. Landfield & S. A. Deadwyler, Eds.), New York, Alan R. Liss, in press.

[8] Collingridge, G. L. & Bliss, T. V. P. (1987) Trends in Neurosci. 10:288-293.

[9] Levy, W. B & Burger, B. (1987) Soc. Neurosci. Abstr. 13:in press.

[10] Burger, B. & Levy, W. B (1987) Soc. Neurosci. Abstr. 13:in press.

[11] Levy, W. B & Steward, O. (1983) Neuroscience 8:799-808.

Primed Burst Potentiation: Lasting Synaptic Plasticity Invoked by Physiologically Patterned Stimulation

G. M. Rose, D. M. Diamond, K. Pang, and T. V. Dunwiddie

Medical Research (151), VAMC and Department of Pharmacology,
UCHSC Denver, Colorado 80220, USA

Primed burst potentiation combines two prominent aspects of hippocampal physiology, complex-spike discharge and theta rhythm, to produce lasting increases in evoked responses recorded in area CA1. This effect is seen in both the *in vitro* slice preparation and in the intact hippocampus of unanesthetized rats.

Long-term potentiation (LTP), a lasting increase in synaptic efficacy seen following high-frequency stimulation, has been extensively studied as a mnemonic model. However, a major conceptual difficulty in relating LTP to an endogenous mechanism for memory formation is that the parameters commonly used for its induction are well beyond the normal physiological firing range of hippocampal neurons: usually 50-400 stimuli, delivered at frequencies of 100-400 Hz, are employed (Teyler and Discenna, 1984). While hippocampal pyramidal cells are known to discharge in "complex-spikes", consisting of several action potentials at frequencies greater that 100 Hz, groups of 3 or 4 action potentials are most commonly seen (Suzuki and Smith, 1985); continuous high frequency discharge is only observed under experimentally-induced or pathological conditions. We considered the possibility that the threshold for the induction of LTP might be reduced if the pattern of stimulation more accurately reflected normal neuronal firing.

Experiments were conducted using the *in vitro* hippocampal slice preparation, as well as in unanesthetized, freely moving rats. For the slice experiments, Ca^{++} and Mg^{++} levels were both 2.5 mM, and the slices were kept entirely submerged in the perfusion medium. For the chronic studies, animals were anesthetized with secobarbital and a stimulating electrode was implanted in the ventral hippocampal commissure. Contralateral to the stimulation site, a microdrive base was located over the dorsal hippocampus. One to two weeks following the surgery, a miniature microdrive was attached to the base to allow the placement of a recording electrode in the CA1 pyramidal cell layer. Responses of the pyramidal neurons were recorded following electrical stimulation of the commissural/associational afferents to their apical dendrites. For both the slice and intact animal studies, stimulus intensities were adjusted to evoke baseline responses consisting of a positive field EPSP and a small (0.5-2.0 mv) population spike. Normal stimulus frequency was once per minute. A computer was used to digitize, automatically measure and continuously display changes in the evoked response.

Our basic finding is illustrated in Figure 1. A patterned train of only 5 stimuli (a priming pulse followed 170 ms later by a burst consisting of 4 pulses at 100 Hz) was sufficient to induce a long lasting increase in the magnitude of the population spike evoked by subsequent single stimuli. Accompanying changes in the slope of the positive field EPSP were usually, but not always, observed. Other patterns of 5-pulse stimulus presentation (e.g., reversing the order of the priming pulse and the burst; Rose and Dunwiddie, 1986), or the delivery of up to 10 pulses at 100 Hz, did not produce lasting effects.

H.L. Haas   G. Buzsàki (Eds.)
Synaptic Plasticity in the Hippocampus
© Springer-Verlag Berlin Heidelberg 1988

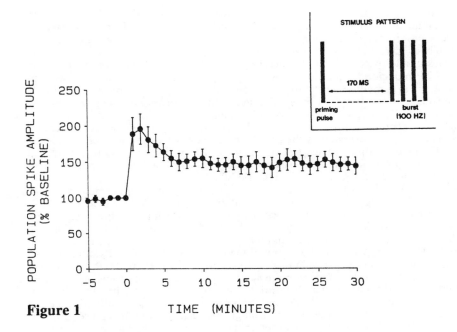

Figure 1   TIME (MINUTES)

The most effective interval between the priming pulse and the subsequent burst was approximately 140-170 ms; intervals less than 100 ms or greater than 500 ms had no long-term effect on population spike amplitude. A total of at least 4 stimuli (1 + 3) was necessary to elicit a lasting increase in the population spike; from this threshold, the magnitude of the change was proportional to the number of stimuli delivered following the priming pulse (up to 10). Although smaller in amplitude, primed burst (PB) potentiation was similar in both timecourse and duration to LTP induced by 100 Hz/1 sec stimulation. However, unlike LTP in area CA1, PB potentiation could be induced heterosynaptically if the priming pulse and subsequent train were delivered to different dendritic fields; in these cases, only the burst-stimulated input was potentiated. When the effectiveness of homosynaptic versus heterosynaptic PB trains was compared, no difference in the average increase in population spike amplitude was seen. Antidromic activation of the pyramidal cells was not effective as a priming pulse.

In the intact hippocampus, PB potentiation was not quite as reliably evoked as in the slice preparation (17/26 attempts, versus 31/40 attempts in the slice), although their average amplitudes were similar (approximately 150% of control 30 minutes after initiation). In addition, the presence of anesthesia was detrimental to the induction of PB potentiation. In animals anesthetized with either urethane or secobarbital, the default stimulus parameters (1 + 4 pulses) never resulted in an enhancement of the evoked response. However, increasing the duration of the burst to 10 pulses was consistently effective.

Several lines of evidence demonstrated that the potentiating effects of PB and LTP trains were not additive. First, if several sequential LTP (100 Hz/1 sec) trains were delivered at 10 minute intervals, the increment in population spike amplitude became smaller with each succeeding train. (The stimulus voltage was reduced between the trains such that the population spike was reduced to its initial amplitude.) After 3-5 trains, LTP was "saturated", i.e. no further increase in the response could be evoked. A PB train administered at this point caused a further increase in the population spike in only 1 of 9 cases; on average, no significant change was observed. In addition, PB trains delivered prior to the LTP-inducing stimulus reduced the effect of the LTP train in an incremental manner. Thus, on average, LTP induced after a single PB train was smaller than that seen without a preceding PB train, and was still smaller if 2 or 3 PB-inducing trains had been given before LTP stimulation.

The lack of additivity between the increases in population spike amplitude following PB- and LTP-inducing stimulation trains suggests that the two phenomena share the same underlying mechanism. Pharmacological investigations of primed burst potentiation also support this idea. Perfusion of hippocampal slices with either phencyclidine (PCP; 10 μM) or 2-amino-5-phosphonovalerate (AP5; 50 μM), which are both NMDA receptor antagonists, had little effect upon baseline stimulus-evoked responses. (A slight depression of the population spike was sometimes seen following AP5 application; in these cases, the stimulus voltage was increased to return the response to pre-drug amplitude). However, PCP and AP5, at concentrations which were shown to prevent LTP, also blocked the PB effect.

In sum, two well-known physiological characteristics of the hippocampal neurons, complex-spike discharge and rhythmic activity at approximately 6-7 Hz (theta rhythm), can be combined into a pattern of electrical stimulation which is capable of eliciting a long term increase in the amplitude of the CA1 population spike evoked by commissural/associational afferent stimulation. This phenomenon, termed primed burst potentiation, appears to have many of the characteristics of LTP, and may also share the same underlying mechanism. However, in contrast to LTP, our results demonstrate that long-term changes in the strength of hippocampal connections may be achieved using stimulation which mimics normal afferent activity. In addition, determining the mechanism of PB potentiation should be greatly simplified since the phenomenon is entirely dependent upon a single, but critical, stimulus pulse. Finally, unlike LTP, PB potentiation can be induced in the target neuron by the cooperative, but temporally dependent, activity of separate afferents; in this regard, PB potentiation is perhaps the worthier candidate for a mechanism underlying associative memory.

Supported by the Veterans Administration Medical Research Service and USPHS grant DA 02702.

References

Rose, G.M., Dunwiddie, T.V.: Induction of hippocampal long-term potentiation using physiologically patterned stimulation. Neurosci. Lett. **69**, 244-248 (1986)

Suzuki, S.S., Smith, G.K.: Burst characteristics of hippocampal complex spike cells in the awake rat. Exp. Neurol. **89**, 90-95 (1985)

Teyler, T.J., Discenna, P.: Long-term potentiation as a candidate mnemonic device. Brain Res. Rev. **7**, 15-28 (1984)

Collective Behaviors of the Hippocampal Slice – Epileptic and Nonepileptic

R. D. Traub, R. Miles, and R. K. S. Wong

IBM T.J. Watson Research Center, Yorktown Heights, NY 10598, USA and Department of Neurology, Columbia University, New York, NY 10032, USA

In this note, we shall review some experimental and computer-simulation results on neuronal population behaviors of the CA3 region *in vitro*. We are particularly interested in the phenomenon of synchronized neuronal bursting. Under what conditions can synchronization develop? Is disinhibition required? Can synchronization develop locally, and if so, what determines whether and at what velocity a synchronized event will propagate? These questions are important for understanding epilepsy, for the light they shed on synaptic actions and connectivity, and as a foundation for the investigation of experience-induced plasticity (since local tetanic stimulation leads to the development of synchrony within the tetanized region (Miles and Wong, in prep.)).

Given that individual CA3 neurons can burst in isolation (13), the problem of synchronized bursting clearly involves an analysis of how pyramidal cells interact with each other. Our first model consisted of a set of neurons connected only by excitatory synapses (12), without any synaptic inhibition. This model was directed toward experiments in which synchronized bursts occur following blockade of one form of GABAergic inhibition with convulsant agents such as penicillin, bicuculline or picrotoxin (PTX). We were guided by these observations: 1) block of synaptic activity (but not with zero-calcium solutions) abolished synchronized discharges while individual cells retained the ability to burst, suggesting that a threshold degree of synaptic transmission was required; 2) highly localized stimuli could evoke a full synchronized discharge, with a latency to field potential onset of tens of ms, implying that synapses should be powerful enough for bursting to propagate from cell to cell (subsequently verified experimentally (4)). With this model, we could reproduce the experimental observations, and predicted that intracellular stimulation of one cell should evoke synchrony, a finding that holds for at least some neurons (2). This model can be further checked, since it is possible to estimate the probability of excitatory interconnections and the size of unitary EPSPs. Using plausible values for these parameters, the model generates a synaptic conductance at the height of synchrony (9) consistent with experimental estimates (1).

When slow inhibition is included in this model, synchrony can still develop, provided there is an appropriate balance between build-up of excitation (depending critically on the number of cells contacted by any given pyramidal cell) and the long-latency for slow inhibition to reach levels sufficient to prevent burst propagation (9). With the synaptic connectivity (connection probability 1% to 2% in regions of the transverse slice containing about 1000 neurons (4)), and IPSP onset kinetics (peak at 50 ms or more after a stimulus) actually observed in CA3, this appropriate balance does exist.

By dual intracellular recording, it has been possible to characterize unitary IPSPs in the CA3 region (3). These events occur with brief latency after a single action potential and decay with time constant close to the membrane time constant. As PTX is washed into the bath, several interesting things happen: the probability of observing polysynaptic excitatory interactions rises,

H.L. Haas   G. Buzsàki (Eds.)
Synaptic Plasticity in the Hippocampus
© Springer-Verlag Berlin Heidelberg 1988

as does the effect that stimulating one cell has on the entire system. Thus, stimulating one cell may induce first in another cell either an IPSP or no apparent potential, then an EPSP, then a double EPSP, and then an EPSP followed by a burst (5). During spontaneous activity, synchronized EPSPs begin to emerge as inhibition is blocked; these increase in amplitude and finally develop into synchronized bursts (5). Synchronized recurring synaptic potentials have been observed in other preparations as well (6-8).

We included in our randomly connected model a subpopulation of neurons whose postsynaptic action was a rapidly decaying inhibitory conductance similar to that studied experimentally (9). We "titrated" the level of the inhibitory conductance, corresponding to various degrees of inhibitory blockade by PTX. One functional effect of inhibition is to limit the propagation of bursting from one neuron to another (5). Propagation of bursting from a stimulated cell may occur to at least some other cells at *any* inhibitory strength simply because the inhibitory cells activated by the stimulated cell may not, in a random network, inhibit all the pyramidal cells excited by the stimulated cell. As inhibition is progressively blocked, activity can percolate further into the system, on a time scale of tens of ms, eliciting EPSPs, IPSPs, and sometimes action potentials or bursts, downstream. In particular, as inhibition is progressively blocked, some downstream cells display the same sequence of EPSP, double EPSP, etc. described above (9).

Similar ideas underlie the behavior of the model during its spontaneous activity (11). Here, burst propagation is limited not only by synaptic inhibition but also by intrinsic refractoriness in cells which have burst recently. At levels of inhibition greater than would allow full synchronized discharges, the model generates periodic "miniature" synchronized events, with interevent periods of several hundred ms. As a small cluster of cells discharges in phase, cells postsynaptic to the cluster (such cells forming a significant fraction of the total population) will in turn exhibit periodic synchronized synaptic potentials - just as happens experimentally. The detailed mechanism by which miniature synchronized events are produced in this model, and mechanisms determining their period of recurrence, are discussed elsewhere (11).

Finally, we considered the question as to whether networks of hippocampal neurons are truly randomly connected on a global scale. It appears that, at least along the longitudinal axis, connections are more likely to occur near to a presynaptic cell than far away. When a longitudinal slice bathed in PTX is stimulated at one end, a synchronized discharge first develops at the stimulated end and then propagates (as measured by either intra- or extracellular potentials) along the slice at 0.1 to 0.25 m/s. In a normal medium, a propagating synchronized discharge does not occur, but synaptic potentials occur up to 2 to 3 mm from the stimulus, whose latency increases with distance from the stimulus. Axon conduction velocity measured in this way is 0.45 to 0.6 m/s, significantly faster than the propagation velocity of the synchronized discharge (10). Such observations can be reproduced in a model wherein excitatory synaptic connection probability falls off with distance, but not in a globally random model. Excitatory connections are thus localized, at least in a statistical sense. Our model furthermore makes two predictions, both in agreement with experiment. 1) when a band of cells across the slice is strongly hyperpolarized (corresponding to GABA application), synchrony is blocked locally but reappears distal to the hyperpolarized region after a delay; 2) in the presence of a small degree of synaptic inhibition, small amplitude, partially synchronized events occur that propagate at velocities *lower* than for events occurring during complete inhibitory blockade (10).

Preliminary simulations are now underway to examine the effects of inhibition in an extended model with localized excitatory connectivity. These, together with experiments on localized stimulation in the presence of inhibition, and on synchrony in a region of focal blockade of inhibition with PTX, suggest that inhibitory connectivity is also localized, perhaps more so even than excitatory connectivity. Such a model can be used to aid in the analysis of ongoing work on post-tetanic synaptic plasticity.

References

1. JOHNSTON, D. and BROWN, T.H. Giant synaptic potential hypothesis for epileptiform activity. *Science, NY.* 211: 294-297, 1981.

2. MILES, R. and WONG, R.K.S. Single neurones can influence synchronized population discharge in the CA3 region of the guinea pig hippocampus. *Nature* 306: 371-373, 1983.

3. MILES, R. and WONG, R.K.S. Unitary inhibitory synaptic potentials in the guinea-pig hippocampus *in vitro. J. Physiol., Lond.* 356: 97-113, 1984.

4. MILES, R. and WONG, R.K.S. Excitatory synaptic interactions between CA3 neurones in the guinea pig hippocampus. *J. Physiol., Lond.* 373: 397-418, 1986.

5. MILES, R. and WONG, R.K.S. Inhibitory control of local excitatory synaptic circuits in the guinea pig hippocampus. *J. Physiol., Lond.* in press.

6. SCHNEIDERMAN, J.H. Low concentrations of penicillin reveal rhythmic, synchronous synaptic potentials in hippocampal slice. *Brain Res.* 398: 231-241, 1986.

7. SCHWARTZKROIN, P.A. and HAGLUND, M.M. Spontaneous rhythmic synchronous activity in epileptic human and normal monkey temporal lobe. *Epilepsia* 27: 523-533, 1986.

8. SCHWARTZKROIN, P.A. and KNOWLES, W.D. Intracellular study of human epileptic cortex: *in vitro* maintenance of epileptiform activity. *Science* 223: 709-712, 1984.

9. TRAUB, R.D., MILES, R. and WONG, R.K.S. Models of synchronized hippocampal bursts in the presence of inhibition. I. Single population events. *J. Neurophysiol.* in press.

10. TRAUB, R.D., MILES, R. and WONG, R.K.S. Studies of propagating epileptic events in the longitudinal hippocampal slice. *Soc. Neurosci. Abstr.* in press.

11. TRAUB, R.D., MILES, R., WONG, R.K.S., SCHULMAN, L.S. and SCHNEIDERMAN, J.H. Models of synchronized hippocampal bursts in the presence of inhibition. II. Ongoing spontaneous population events. *J. Neurophysiol.*

12. TRAUB, R.D. and WONG, R.K.S. Cellular mechanism of neuronal synchronization in epilepsy. *Science, NY.* 216: 745-747, 1982.

13. WONG, R.K.S., MILES, R. and TRAUB, R.D. Local circuit interactions in synchronization of cortical neurones. *J. Exp. Biol.* 112: 169-178, 1984.

Are Nerve Growth Factors Involved in Long-Term Synaptic Potentiation in the Hippocampus and Spatial Memory?

B. R. Sastry, S. S. Chirwa, P. B. Y. May, H. Maretić, G. Pillai, E. Y. H. Kao, and S. D. Sidhu

Neuroscience Research Laboratory, Department of Pharmacology and Therapeutics, Faculty of Medicine, The University of British Columbia, Vancouver, BC V6T 1W5, Canada

Growth factors released by tetanic stimulations of the cerebral cortex and the hippocampus, appear to be involved in long-term synaptic potentiation and in spatial memory. It, therefore, appears that LTP and spatial memory in adults may very well be expressions of a continuation of certain aspects of the developing nervous system.

Nerve growth factor (NGF), which facilitates the development of the nervous system (levi-Montalcini and Angeletti, 1968), is present in the hippocampus and is known to be released following injury to hippocampal pathways (Crutcher and Collins, 1986; Nieto-Sampedro and Cotman, 1985). NGF is believed to be released from the postsynaptic neurons and taken up by the presynaptic terminals; it causes sprouting of boutons and brings about biochemical changes in the presynaptic terminals (Hendry et al., 1974; Springer and Loy, 1985). High frequency activation of hippocampal afferents causes a subsequent long-term potentiation (LTP) of synaptic transmission (Bliss and Lømo, 1973) between these inputs and the pyramidal neurons. The mechanisms involved in the induction and maintenance of this potentiation are of significant interest to neuroscientists because of its presumed involvement in learning and memory, two of the most important functions of the brain. A depolarization of the CA_1 neurons in association with presynaptic activity and a patterned stimulation of hippocampal inputs in association with theta rhythm are both thought to be necessary for LTP (Kelso et al., 1986; Larson and Lynch, 1986; Sastry et al., 1986; Wigström et al., 1986). How a cooperation between the activity in the presynaptic terminal and a depolarization of the postsynaptic neuron can lead to LTP is not clear. As one of the possibilities, we previously suggested that the postsynaptic depolarization induces the release of a chemical which acts on the stimulated presynaptic terminal to cause further changes leading to LTP (Sastry et al., 1986; May et al., 1987; also see Eccles, 1983). During LTP synaptic rearrangement, alterations in the shape of the synaptic components, as well as an enhancement in transmitter release were suggested to take place (Desmond and Levy, 1981; Fifkova and Van Harreveld, 1977; Lee et al., 1980; Lynch and Baudry, 1984; Skrede and Malthe-Sørenssen, 1981; Voronin, 1983). Since NGF is believed to be released from the postsynaptic cells and is known to act on the presynaptic terminals to induce biochemical as well as morphological changes, we examined whether growth factors are involved in LTP and short-term spatial memory.

In rabbits anaesthetized with halothane, cylindrical cups were positioned on the neocortical surface. A stimulating electrode was placed on the cortical surface through the cup. The cups were filled every 5 min with 0.1 ml of the medium (used for perfusing the hippocampal slices). A total of 2 ml of the medium was collected from each rabbit without stimulating the cortical

H. L. Haas   G. Buzsàki (Eds.)
Synaptic Plasticity in the Hippocampus
© Springer-Verlag Berlin Heidelberg 1988

surface (unstimulated neocortical sample, UNS). After this collection, 4 mls were collected while the neocortex was tetanized (tetanized neocortical sample, TNS) (50 Hz for 5 s, every 5 min).

In guinea pig hippocampal slices, population spikes (PS) were recorded from the CA$_1$ and CA$_3$ cell body layers in response to stratum radiatum and mossy fibre stimulation, respectively. TNS (2 ml), when applied on the hippocampal slice, produced LTP (165-650%, n=12) of the CA$_1$ PS that was evoked at 0.2 Hz (see Fig. 1). Neither UNS (2 ml, n=12) nor a preheated and cooled TNS (2 ml, heated at 85 C for 30 min, n=10) had a significant potentiating action on the PS. We previously reported similar effects by samples collected from guinea pig hippocampus (Chirwa and Sastry, 1987). Saccharin reportedly interferes with the binding of NGF to its "receptors" and decreases neurite growth (Ishi, 1982). We, therefore, examined the effects of Na saccharin on the induction of LTP. Na saccharin (10 mM; 10-15 min) blocked the induction of LTP (400 Hz, 200 pulses to the input) in CA$_1$ (n=9) and CA$_3$ (n=5) areas. In the same slices, a subsequent tetanus in the absence of the drug resulted in LTP (PS, 20 min post-tetanus: 125-638% in CA$_1$, 7 of 9; 130-200% in CA$_3$, 5 of 5). The drug did not have a significant effect on the membrane potential, input resistance, and the depolarization of CA$_1$ neurons induced by 0.025-0.075 mM N-methyl-DL-aspartate (n=6). If TNS was applied in the presence of Na saccharin (10 mM), the neocortical sample did not induce LTP (n=4). Tetanic stimulations of stratum radiatum (50 Hz, 10 pulses) that induced only a short-term potentiation (of the weak CA$_1$ population EPSP) in the control medium containing 0.01-0.1 mM picrotoxin, induced LTP (population EPSP 20 min post-tetanus: 135-214%) if the same tetanus was given during a 5-10 min application of NGF (from <u>Vipera labetina</u>, 0.05 mg; n=4). These actions were blocked if NGF was given in the presence of 10 mM Na saccharin (n=6). NGF did not produce a potentiation of the CA$_1$ PS if applied during the absence of stratum radiatum stimulation. The agent had inconsistent effects if applied during 0.2 Hz stimulation of the input.

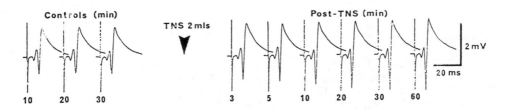

Fig. 1. LTP of the guinea pig hippocampal CA$_1$ PS produced by the application of TNS (2 mls).

Pheochromocytoma cells (PC-12) were grown in culture and incubated with UNS or preheated TNS or TNS and the growth of the neurites monitored. Cells incubated with TNS showed significantly greater neurite growth than the others (n=6).

Male Wistar rats (100-125 g) were trained to find a platform hidden in a water bath (as described by Morris <u>et al.</u>, 1986) in less than 45 s. If Na saccharin (6 mg) was injected underneath the dura on the cerebral cortex of the previously trained rats (for 4 days), they did not locate the platform in 180 s for 1-2 days (n=10) while the control rats injected with the vehicle continued to improve their performance (n=10).

The results indicate that NGF or related growth factors could, indeed, be released from the hippocampus as well as from the neocortex by tetanic stimulation and that they could induce LTP. We also show that Na saccharin, a drug that is known to interfere with the binding of NGF to its "receptors" and to decrease the development of neurites, blocks the induction of LTP in guinea pigs and interrupts spatial memory in rats. As to how trophic factors induce synaptic potentiation is unclear. Perhaps, a depolarization of the postsynaptic neurons, that occurs during the tetanic stimulation of the hippocampal afferents, and theta rhythm cause a release of the growth factors through as yet unknown mechanisms. The peptide then interacts with NGF receptors of active (and not quiescent) presynaptic terminals (and/or subsynaptic dendritic membranes) and brings about subsequent changes needed for LTP (eg., changes in the synaptic structure, synaptic rearrangement, alterations in the dendritic morphology, enhancement of transmitter release, etc.). It is possible that the exogenously applied NGF is different from the endogenous trophic factor and, therefore, had weak effects when applied during low frequency stimulation.

Since Alzheimer's patients have problems with memory and learning, the possibility that in these individuals either the trophic factor is not released during learning or that the actions of the peptide are interfered with (see Hefti and Weiner, 1986) needs to be examined. If the release of NGF by intense neuronal activity is a common feature of various areas in the nervous system, it would be important to determine if the growth factor is involved in improving the quality of synaptic transmission and, therefore, the quality of brain function in general.

In conclusion, growth factors that contribute to the early development of the nervous system seem to play a role in LTP and spatial memory in the adult animal. In this regard LTP and spatial memory may very well be expressions of a continuation of certain aspects of this early development.

These studies were supported by a grant from the Canadian MRC to BRS. SSC is a WHO fellow. EYHK and SDS are supported by NSERC of Canada.

References

Bliss, TVP & Lømo, T (1973) J. Physiol. (Lond.) 232: 331-356.
Chirwa, SS & Sastry, BR (1987) J. Physiol. (Lond.) 386: 29P.
Crutcher, KA & Collins, F (1986) Brain Res. 399: 383-389.
Desmond, NL & Levy, WB (1981) Anat. Rec. 199: 68A-69A.
Eccles, JC (1983) Neuroscience 10: 1071-1081.
Fifkova, E & Van Harreveld, A (1977) J, Neurophysiol. 6: 211-230.
Hefti, F & Weiner, WJ (1986) Ann. Neurol. 20: 275-281.
Hendry, IA, Stokel, K, Thoenen, H & Iversen, LL (1974) Brain Res. 68: 103-121.
Ishi, DN (1982) Cancer Res. 42: 429-432.
Kelso, SR, Ganong, AH & Brown, TH (1986) Proc. Natl. Acad. Sci. USA 83: 5326-5330.
Larson, J. & Lynch G. (1986) Science 232: 985-988.
Lee, KS, Schottler, F, Oliver, M & Lynch, G (1980) J. Neurophysiol. 44: 247-258.
Levi-Montalcini, R & Angeletti, PU (1968) Physiol. rev. 48: 534-569.
Lynch, G & Baudry, M (1984) Science 224: 1057-1063.
May, PBY, Goh, JW & Sastry, BR (1987) Synapse 1: 273-278.
Morris, RGM, Anderson, E, Lynch, GS & Baudry, M (1986) Nature 319: 744-746.
Nieto-Sampedio, M & Cotman, CW (1985) In: Synaptic Plasticity Ed. CW

Cotman, Guilford Press, NY, PP 407-455.

Sastry, BR., Goh, JW & Auyeung, A (1986) Science 232: 988-990.

Skrede, KK & Malthe-Sørenssen, D (1981) Brain Res. 208: 436-441.

Springer, JE & Loy, R (1985) Brain Res. Bull. 15: 629-634.

Voronin, LL (1983) Neuroscience 10: 1051-1069.

Wigström, H, Gustafsson, B, Huang, Y.-Y & Abraham, WC (1986) Acta Physiol. Scand. 126: 317-319.

Molecular Mechanisms
of Long-Term Potentiation

Intracellular Injection of Protein Kinase C Causes Changes Similar to Long-Term Potentiation

G.-Y. Hu[1], Ø. Hvalby[2], S. I. Walaas[3], K. Albert[3], P. Greengard[3], and P. Andersen[2]

[1]Department of Pharmacology III, Shanghai Institute of Materia Medica, Academia Sinica, Shanghai, China
[2]Institute of Neurophysiology, University of Oslo, Oslo, Norway
[3]Laboratory of Molecular and Cellular Neuroscience, The Rockefeller University, New York, NY, USA

Protein kinases are involved in many neuronal changes induced by activity. Application of phorbol ester causes changes in transmission across certain hippocampal synapses similar to those seen during LTP (Malenka et al., 1986). For this reason, we have injected purified protein kinase C (PK-C) in CA1 hippocampal cells and tested its effect on synaptic activation by afferents in stratum radiatum. The activity of the kinase was tested biochemically before and after the injection.

Injection of active PK-C caused a marked increase in the probability of firing to a constant stimulus (p<0.01) starting after about 5 min and lasting for the observation period of 30-35 min. Simultaneously, there was reduced spike latency and increased EPSP amplitude, the normalized EPSP reached about 1.5 times the control level (n=9). There were also a small and delayed hyperpolarization, and a slowly developing reduction of the size of the slow afterhyperpolarization, but no significant change in the soma input resistance. Injection of the enzyme itself was sufficient to create these changes without extra activators.

In control experiments with inactive kinase (n=4), there was no change in the parameters mentioned above, except a moderate hyperpolarization.

In conclusion, injection of active, but not inactive protein kinase C, gives the same changes as seen during long-term potentiation. However, the long-lasting effect seen need not necessarily be identical to LTP, but could be explained by the persistence of the activated enzyme.

Malenka, R.C., Madison, D.V. and Nicoll, R.A. (1986). Nature 321: 175-177.

H.L. Haas G. Buzsàki (Eds.)
Synaptic Plasticity in the Hippocampus
© Springer-Verlag Berlin Heidelberg 1988

On the Mechanism of Increased Transmitter Release in LTP: Measurements of Calcium Concentration and Phosphatidylinositol Turnover in CA3 Synaptosomes

M. A. LYNCH, M. P. CLEMENTS, M. L. ERRINGTON, and T. V. P. BLISS

National Institute for Medical Research, Mill Hill, London NW7 IAA, United Kingdom

The concentration of free calcium in synaptosomes prepared from hippocampal tissue which had been potentiated in vivo was increased compared
to control tissue. Potentiated tissue was also associated with an
increase in inositol phospholipid hydrolysis. These findings are
discussed as possible mechanisms underlying the increase in transmitter
release associated with long-term potentiation.

There is now convincing evidence from many laboratories that both pre and
postsynaptic mechanisms play a role in the induction and/or maintenance of
LTP. In our laboratory, we have demonstrated that the maintenance of LTP
is associated with an increase in release of neurotransmitter – evidence
which is now strongly supported by recent quantal release data (see papers
by both Voronin and Yamamoto, this volume). Since Turner, Baimbridge and
Miller (1982) reported that exposure of hippocampal slices to a high
concentration of calcium induced a form of LTP, the requirement for calcium
in the induction and maintenance of LTP has been firmly established, though
its precise role is still unclear. More recently, the likelihood that
activation of protein kinase C was involved was strengthened by the
observation that phorbol esters also induce a form of LTP (Malenka, Madison
and Nicholl, 1986). We have reported that both calcium and activation of
protein kinase C also modulate glutamate release (Lynch and Bliss, 1986;
1986a) and so we decided to investigate (1) the concentration of free
calcium in synaptosomes prepared from control and potentiated hippocampus
and (2) inositol phospholipid hydrolysis, which would lead to activation of
protein kinase C, in control and potentiated tissue.

Male Sprague-Dawley rats were anaesthetized with urethane and LTP was
induced in the dentate gyrus by high-frequency stimulation of the
perforant path or in area CA3 by stimulating the commissural input to CA3
pyramidal cells. Control animals received the same total number of
stimuli but without the high-frequency train. Forty minutes after the
train the animals were killed, the dentate gyrus or area CA3 dissected out
and slices or synaptosomes (P_2) prepared as previously described (Lynch and
Bliss, 1986a). To measure intrasynaptosomal calcium concentration,
aliquots of the P_2 synaptosomal preparations were loaded with the
calcium-sensitive dye, Indo 1, and the calcium concentration was measured
by fluorescence. Inositol phospholipid hydrolysis was examined in slices
or synaptosomes from control and potentiated hippocampi according to a
method previously described by others (Brown, Kendall and Nahorsky, 1984).
Briefly, tissue was labelled with ^{3}H inositol by incubating in the
presence of LiCl at 37°C. In some experiments glutamate (10^{-3}M) was added
during the incubation period. The reaction was stopped by addition of
ice-cold chloroform, methanol and water and labelling of inositol
phosphates and phosphoinositides by ^{3}H inositol was assessed in the
aqueous and organic phases respectively.

H. L. Haas   G. Buzsàki (Eds.)
Synaptic Plasticity in the Hippocampus
© Springer-Verlag Berlin Heidelberg 1988

Labelling of inositol phosphates by ^{3}H inositol in slices and synaptosomes prepared from potentiated tissue was significantly increased compared to control tissue (Fig. 1). Separation of inositol phosphates into inositol monophosphate (InsP), inositol bisphosphate (InsP$_2$) and inositol trisphosphate (InsP$_3$) showed that there was an increase in labelling of all inositol phosphates associated with potentiation but that in slices only the labelling of InsP reached statistical significance while in synaptosomes labelling of InsP$_2$ and InsP$_3$ were significantly enhanced. These findings suggest that there is an increase in inositol phospholipid hydrolysis associated with LTP. The enhancement occurs in synaptosomes, which are considered to be largely presynaptic, and slices which contain both pre and postsynaptic components. We confirmed that labelling of ^{3}H inositol in the synaptosomal preparation was predominantly to presynaptic elements by further fractionation of P$_2$. Aliquots of labelled P$_2$ were added to a Percoll gradient and separated into a membrane fraction, a mitochondrial fraction and a pure synaptosomal fraction. ^{3}H inositol label was recovered mainly from the synaptosomal fraction (78%) and the remainder was associated with the membrane and mitochondrial fractions (11% in each case). Glutamate mimics the effect of potentiation in control slices but fails to do so in potentiated slices and this result is consistent with the idea that glutamate release, which is increased in LTP (Bliss, Douglas, Errington and Lynch, 1986), maximally stimulates the effect following potentiation. Since glutamate is without effect in synaptosomes, it is likely that the glutamate-induced increase in inositol phosphate labelling is postsynaptic in origin. In contrast to the changes observed in labelling of inositol phosphates by ^{3}H inositol, labelling of phosphoinositides remained unchanged following potentiation (Fig. 1).

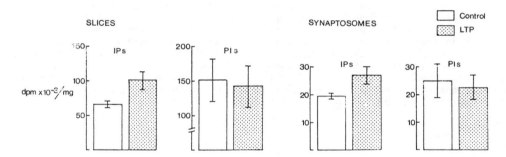

Fig. 1 Labelling of inositol phosphates (IPs) and phosphoinositides (PIs) by ^{3}H inositol in slices and synaptosomes obtained from control or potentiated tissue. There was a significant increase in ^{3}H inositol labelling of inositol phosphates but not phosphoinositides associated with LTP (p < 0.05). Results (means ± SEM; n = 8) presented are from experiments on area CA3: similar results were obtained in the dentate gyrus.

Synaptosomal calcium concentration measured using the fluorescent dye Indo 1 was between 150 and 250 nM in both dentate and CA3. There was an increase in the concentration of calcium in synaptosomes prepared from potentiated tissue compared to control tissue in both areas (Fig. 2).

The increase in calcium concentration observed following potentiation could arise from either intracellular or extracellular sources. Since InsP$_3$ was also increased in potentiated tissue, we considered that it might increase release from some intracellular store in this tissue as it has

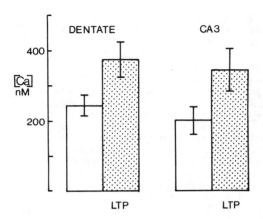

Fig. 2. Concentration of calcium in synaptosomes prepared from control (clear histograms) and potentiated (hatched histograms) tissue of dentate gyrus and area CA3. Results are expressed in nM and given as the mean ± SEM (n = 8 in each case). Calcium concentration is significantly greater in synaptosomes obtained from potentiated tissue compared to control in both hippocampal areas (p < 0.05).

been shown to do in many others (Berridge and Irvine, 1984). To investigate this possibility, Ins(1,4,5)P$_3$ was incorporated into synaptosomes during their preparation, the synaptosomes loaded with Indo 1 and calcium concentration measured as described above. The calcium concentration in synaptosomes to which Ins(1,4,5)P$_3$ had been added was significantly greater than that in untreated synaptosomes (Fig 3). However, the effect of Ins(1,4,5)P$_3$ in synaptosomes prepared from potentiated tissue was much reduced compared to control. This may indicate that Ins(1,4,5)P$_3$ stimulates release of calcium from intracellular stores following potentiation thereby accounting for the partial occlusion observed. It should be noted that in these experiments we confirmed our earlier observation that there was an increase in calcium concentration in synaptosomes prepared from potentiated tissue. In separate experiments we confirmed the findings of Agoston and Kuhnt (1986) showing that there was an increase in calcium influx associated with LTP (results not shown). These results indicate therefore that the increase in calcium concentration demonstrated in LTP is probably a result of influx from the extracellular medium combined with release from intracellular stores.

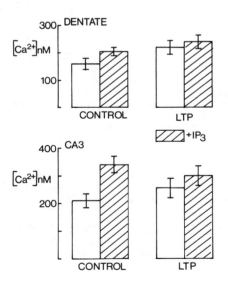

Fig. 3. Effect of inositol(1,4,5) trisphosphate (IP$_3$, hatched histograms) on synaptosomal calcium concentration in preparations obtained from control and potentiated dentate gyrus and area CA3. Results are expressed in nM and are the means ± SEM of 6 observations. IP$_3$ significantly increased calcium concentration in control synaptosomes in both areas (p < 0.05) but the small increase in potentiated synaptosomes failed to reach statistical significance.

We have shown that there is an increase in inositol phospholipid hydrolysis in slices and synaptosomes prepared from potentiated tissue suggesting that both pre and postsynaptic components are involved: our findings are consistent with the idea that glutamate stimulates the postsynaptic change. One consequence of this change would be an increase in formation of diacyl glycerol and therefore activation of protein kinase C, which has been shown to modulate transmitter release (Lynch and Bliss, 1986a) and induce a form of LTP (Malenka et al., 1986). We have also demonstrated that there is an increase in the intrasynaptosomal concentration of calcium in potentiated tissue compared to control tissue. It is likely that the increase in calcium concentration derives from both intracellular and extracellular sources since $Ins(1,4,5)P_3$, which is increased in potentiated tissue, enhances intracellular calcium release, and calcium influx is increased following potentiation. We propose that the increase in intrasynaptosomal calcium and/or the increase in protein kinase C activation, could contribute to the enhanced transmitter release associated with LTP which we have previously described (Bliss et al., 1986).

Agoston, DV & Kuhnt, U (1986) Exp. Brain Res., 62, 663–668.

Berridge, MJ & Irvine, RF (1984) Nature, 312, 315–321.

Bliss, TVP, Douglas, RM, Errington, ML & Lynch, MA (1986) J. Physiol., 377, 391–408.

Brown, E, Kendall, DA & Nahorsky, SR, (1984) J. Neurochem., 42, 1379–1387.

Lynch, MA & Bliss, TVP (1986) Brain Res. 369, 405–408

Lynch, MA & Bliss, TVP (1986a) Neurosci. Letts., 65, 171–176.

Malenka, RC, Madison, DV & Nicoll, RA (1986) Nature, 319, 774–776.

Turner, RW, Baimbridge, KG & Miller, JJ (1982) Neuroscience, 7, 1411–1416.

Effects of Phorbol Esters on Membrane Currents and Synaptic Efficacy in the Hippocampus

D. V. Madison[1], R. C. Malenka, and R. A. Nicoll

Departments of Pharmacology and Physiology, University of California, San Francisco, CA 94143, USA ([1]present address: Department of Physiology, Yale School of Medicine, New Haven, CT 06510, USA

Application of phorbol esters to hippocampal slices has been shown to enhance synaptic transmission in a way that mimics long term potentiation. These compounds also have effects on a voltage-dependent chloride current that could possibly account for some aspects of this potentiating action.

Second messenger systems serve an important function in controlling the excitability of neurons and other cells through mechanisms involving the modulation of voltage- and calcium-dependent ionic conductances. Cyclic AMP, working through activation of protein kinase A, has been identified as the second messenger for several neurotransmitters. Activation of the calcium- and phospholipid-dependent protein kinase C (PKC) may also have similar actions on neurons. In mammalian brain, PKC activation has been shown to phosphorylate several substrate proteins, one of which may be involved in producing long term potentiation (LTP)[1,2]. We have shown that activation of PKC, with the phorbol ester analogs of diacylglycerol causes a marked increase in excitatory synaptic efficacy that is similar to that seen during long term potentiation (LTP)[3].

Excitatory synaptic potentials (epsps) arising in area CA1 in response to Schaffer collateral stimulation are normally quite stable. In a healthy hippocampal slice preparation, test stimuli delivered over several hours produce synaptic potentials that do not vary in amplitude by more than a few percent. However, when active phorbol esters (PE) are applied to the preparation, these epsps increase in amplitude by up to several hundred percent. This increase in synaptic strength is very similar to that seen during tetanic stimulation-induced long term potentiation. In phorbol ester-induced potentiation, like tetanus-induced LTP, the increase in the epsp can be recorded in the dendritic field potential as well as in the population spike. During both PE- and tetanus-induced potentiation, the latency of the population spike decreases and the relationship between the presynaptic fiber volley and the postsynaptic potential shifts in an identical manner. The PE-induced potentiation is likely to be due to the activation of PKC because application of phorbol esters that are ineffective on PKC do not produce these effects.

To investigate the locus of PE-induced potentiation, we compared the effect of phorbol esters on the extracellular epsp field potential to a similar field potential elicited by pressure application of the excitatory transmitter glutamate, both in the same area of the dendrites. While phorbol ester application markedly increased the population epsp, the glutamate response was unchanged. This suggests that dendritic glutamate sensitivity was not enhanced by PE application and suggests a potential presynaptic locus of the PE-induced potentiation. Indeed it has been demonstrated that PE application

H. L. Haas   G. Buzsàki (Eds.)
Synaptic Plasticity in the Hippocampus
© Springer-Verlag Berlin Heidelberg 1988

causes an increase in potassium stimulated glutamate release suggesting that PE may potentiate synaptic transmission by increasing transmitter release[4].

If PE-induced potentiation and LTP are identical, it should be possible to occlude LTP by pretreatment with phorbol esters. Indeed, when slices were treated with the active forms of PE, tetanic stimulation of the Schaffer collaterals no longer produced LTP. Slices pretreated with inactive phorbol esters potentiated normally. Pretreatment with active PE did not affect the production of short lasting post-tetanic potentiation, indicating that the effect of PE's were confined to the long lasting form of synaptic potentiation.

We have studied the actions of phorbol esters on membrane currents in hippocampal pyramidal cells to gain clues as to the possible mechanism for the potentiating actions of these compounds[5,6]. We, have found that active, but not inactive phorbol esters can block two different membrane currents in CA1 pyramidal neurons. Both the slow calcium-activated potassium conductance (see also ref. 7), and a voltage-dependent chloride current ($I_{Cl(v)}$), are blocked by these compounds. Blockade of the calcium-activated potassium current almost certainly cannot account for the potentiating action of PE because application of 8-bromo cyclic AMP, which selectively blocks this current, does not cause potentiation of synaptic potentials[8]. Blockade of $I_{Cl(v)}$, which is active at resting membrane potentials, may produce effects that could explain in part the potentiating action of PE. A reported postsynaptic correlate of LTP is an increased electrical coupling between the dendritic and somatic regions of pyramidal neurons. This is reflected functionally in the finding that a given sized dendritic synaptic potential will produce a larger somatic population spike than before LTP[9]. A similar phenomenon can be seen during phorbol ester application. Not only will a dendritic synaptic input of a given size produce an enhanced somatic response after PE application, but a fixed dendritic depolarization caused by iontophoresis of glutamate or potassium, can also produce more somatic depolarization after PE administration. Such an enhancement of dendritic-somatic coupling could be accounted for by the blockade of a resting current, such as $I_{Cl(v)}$, and the resulting removal of a resistive shunt between the dendrite and the soma. Since this increase in dendrite to soma electrical coupling could account for only a fraction of the potentiating action of PE, it is also interesting to speculate as to whether the blockade of such a current in presynaptic membranes could account for the bulk of the potentiation caused by these agents.

1. Nelson, R.B. and Routtenberg, A. (1985). **Experimental Neurology 89**, 213-224.
2. Akers, R.F. and Routtenberg, A. (1985). **Brain Research 334**, 147-151.
3. Malenka, R.C., Madison, D.V. and Nicoll, R.A. (1987). **Nature 321**, 175-177.
4. Malenka, R.C., Ayoub, G.S. and Nicoll, R.A. (1987). **Brain Research 403**, 198-203.
5. Malenka, R.C., Madison, D.V., Andrade, R. and Nicoll, R.A. (1986). **Journal of Neuroscience 6**, 475-480.
6. Madison, D.V., Malenka, R.C. and Nicoll, R.A. (1987). **Nature 321**, 695-697.
7. Baraban, J.M., Snyder, S.H. and Alger, B.E. (1985). **Proceedings of the National Academy of Sciences, USA 82**, 2538-2542.
8. Newberry, N.R. and Nicoll, R.A. (1984). **Journal of Physiology 348**, 239-254.
9. Andersen, P., Sundberg, S.H., Sveen, E., Swann, J.W. and Wigström, H. (1980). **Journal of Physiology 302**, 463-482.

Gangliosides and Synaptic Plasticity in the Hippocampus

W. Seifert, A. Wieraszko, and H. Terlau

Department of Neurobiology, Max-Planck-Institut für biophysikalische Chemie,
3400 Göttingen, Federal Republic of Germany

For a long time, it has been suggested that gangliosides might have a functional role in synaptic transmission. We are investigating this hypothesis in the hippocampal slice preparation both for normal transmission and for long-term potentiation (LTP) in the Schaffer Collateral – CA_1 field.

For these studies we have used three different strategies:
– modifying the endogenous ganglioside pattern by treatment of the slice with neuraminidases
– binding or blocking individual gangliosides by addition of cholera toxin, tetanus toxin and monoclonal anti-GM_1-antiserum
– addition of exogenous gangliosides, which are incorporated into the neuronal cell membranes.

The results of our neuraminidase experiments can be summarized as follows: treatment with neuraminidase of *Vibrio cholerae* (NVCh) has no effect on the population spike following low frequency stimulation. Since this enzyme splits off sialic acid from poly-sialo-gangliosides transforming them into the mono-sialo-ganglioside GM_1, it was suggested that polysialo-gangliosides may not be crucially important for glutamatergic transmission. In contrast to this result, the same treatment with NVCh abolished the evoked potential of cholinergic transmission in striatal slices (A.Wieraszko and W.Seifert, 1984, 1986). Thus we concluded that polysialo-gangliosides might be important for cholinergic transmission.
The large increase in the amount of GM_1 in the slices induced by NVCh treatment correlated with an increase in synaptic plasticity following high frequency stimulation (measured 2 min. and 15 min. later). Similar but less pronouced results were obtained by pre-incubation of slices with exogenous GM_1 for 3 hours. Both treatments did not influence he size of the population spike when low frequency stimulation was employed (A.Wieraszko and W.Seifert, 1985).

H.L. Haas   G. Buzsàki (Eds.)
Synaptic Plasticity in the Hippocampus
© Springer-Verlag Berlin Heidelberg 1988

In contrast to the NVCh treatment which did not effect the population spike at low frequence stimulation, the incubation of slices with neuraminidase from *Arthrobacter ureafaciens* (NAu) efficiently abolished the population spike in about 5 hours. Since NAu can eventually split off sialic acid from GM_1, this result seemed to suggest that GM_1 is essential for normal glutamatergic transmission in the hippocampus. But our measurements of the ganglioside pattern following NAu treatment did not support this hypothesis, since due to the concomitant degradation of polysialo-gangliosides by NAu the GM_1 content of the whole slice is actually increased. However, we cannot rule out the possibility that the synaptic content of GM_1 might be reduced. Alternatively the neuraminidase from *Arthrobacter* could also attack sialic acid residues from glycoproteins at the synapse. This in turn might cause the effect on the population spike, while the changes in the ganglioside pattern would be only coincidental rather than causal. At the moment we cannot decide between these possibilities. Experiments with cholera toxin and a monoclonal GM_1-antiserum, which both should bind specifically to GM_1 are in progress and hopefully will help us to clarify this question.

However we can definitly state that the presence of sialic residues – either in gangliosides or glycoproteins – on the surface of the synaptic plasmamembrane is functionally important for the normal transmission in the hippocampal slice: modification by periodate, or binding by ruthenium red, or enzymatic degradation by neuraminidase of *Arthrobacter* (all these treatments effecting sialic residues) will efficiently block synaptic transmission.

Concerning a possible mechanism of action, we favor the idea of gangliosid-calcium complex formation, for which there is some experimental evidence. Since the sialic acid residue is of crucial importance for this process, it seems reasonable that destroying or blocking this part of the ganglioside molecules might lead to functional inactivation of the synapses. This suggestion is supported by experiments with ^{45}Ca in our laboratory which demonstrate that removal of sialic acids by neuraminidase treatment profoundly changes the binding of calcium to the slice (A.Wieraszko and W.Seifert, unpublished).

In a similar way we might expect that the effect of an increased GM_1-content in the slice on synaptic plasticity (LTP at 15 min.) could be due to higher ganglioside-calcium concentration and increased calcium-influx.

On the other hand exogenous addition of GD_1a and GT_1b showed no significant increase in LTP. This can be explained by the relatively small incorporation of gangliosides into the slice as demonstrated by experiments with ^3H-labelled gangliosides. Under standard experimental conditions (3 – 4 hours incubation time, $33°C$, exogenous ganglioside concentration: $70\mu M$) the incorporation corresponds to an increase of 5 – 10 % of the respective ganglioside (H.Terlau and W.Seifert, unpublished).

Another alternative explanation for the effect of increased GM_1-content on synaptic plasticity could be a stimulation of glutamate receptors in the synapses. We have indeed demonstrated a striking increase in glutamate receptor binding to isolated synaptic plasmamembranes following pre-incubation with gangliosides and calcium (M.Hollmann and W.Seifert, 1986).

Whether by calcium-complex formation and resulting changes in calcium-flux or by stimulating the glutamate recepor binding on the postsynaptic membrane, it seems evident that larger increases in the synaptic concentration of individual gangliosides can modulate synaptic plasticity in the hippocampal slice.

References:

1. Wieraszko, A. and Seifert, W., (1985) Brain Res. **345**: 159 – 164.
2. Wieraszko, A. and Seifert, W., (1986) Brain Res. **371**: 305 – 313.
3. Hollmann, M. and Seifert, W., (1986) Neurosc. Letters **65**: 133 – 138.

Long-Term Synaptic Potentiation and Macromolecular Changes in Memory Formation

H. MATTHIES

Institute of Neurobiology and Brain Research, Academy of Sciences of GDR., Leipziger Strasse 44, 3090 Magdeburg, German Democratic Republic

In the course of our investigations on cellular mechanisms of memory formation, we proposed already 15 years ago a three-stage model of information storage in the nervous system, which regards the time course and the sensitiveness of short-term, intermediate and long-term memory to different chemical and physical influences as a reflection of the dynamics and properties of corresponding cellular and molecular mechanisms (Matthies, 1972, 1974, 1982). Accordingly , three regulatory principles of memory formation were distinguished:
- a <u>synaptic regulation</u> of short-term memory in the range of seconds to minutes, mainly presynaptically induced by translocation of electrolyte ions in the course of enhanced synaptic activity, resulting in an increased release and/or synthesis of transmitters.
- a <u>synaptosomal regulation</u> of intermediate memory in the range of minutes to hours, induced pre- and postsynaptically by translocation of ions and by transmitter-receptor interactions, resulting via second messenger systems in conformational changes of existing proteins and subsequent alterations of synaptic efficiency.
- a <u>nuclear regulation</u> of long-term memory developing in the course of hours and lasting more or less permanently, induced by coactivation of different inputs to postsynaptic targets, resulting in second messenger mediated activation of transcriptional, translational and posttranslational steps of macromolecular synthesis and a final functional reconstruction of postsynaptic neurons and/or their connections.
We showed that glycosylation of newly synthesized proteins to complete their functional properties seems to be more critical for the consolidation of a memory trace, than the ribosomal synthesis of polypeptide chains and may be controled by aminergic mediation of motivational, emotional or rewarding influences, thus finally valuating the informations to be stored.
Dopaminergic activation of hippocampal structures, for instance, results in enhanced memory formation as well as in an increased glycosylation of neuronal proteins in vivo and in vitro. Fucosylglycoproteins seem to play a particular role in the formation of permanent traces, the prevention of fucose $1 \rightarrow 2$ galactose coupling in proteo-

H.L. Haas   G. Buzsàki (Eds.)
Synaptic Plasticity in the Hippocampus
© Springer-Verlag Berlin Heidelberg 1988

glycans by pretreatment with 2-deoxygalactose results in a profound amnesia in different learning tasks and species (Jork et al. 1986).
With regard to the assumed role of posttetanic LTP as a mechanism of memory formation, we applied the considerations and experimental results from our learning experiments to an elucidation of this problem. We showed that after acquisition of a conditioned active avoidance with low frequency stimulation of the perforant path as CS, a long-term enhancement slowly develops in the perforant path-granular cell synapses necessarily involved in the conditioning pathway, exhibiting a pronounced contribution of the EPSP component, and occurring only in good learners. Poor learners showed a long-term depression of test potentials, however (Matthies et al. 1986). The acquisition of this conditioned avoidance is accompanied by an increase of glycoprotein synthesis in the hippocampal neurons. However, the fast development of monosynaptic posttetanic LTP was not followed by a corresponding enhancement of glycoprotein synthesis. (Pohle et al. 1987). Comparing the extent of LTP after tetanization, the extent of postconditioning LTP, and the learning ability, the same animals exhibiting a poor posttetanic LTP could also be classified as poor learners and showed a postconditioning long-term depression. The rats with a pronounced posttetanic LTP revealed also high learning scores and a remarkable postconditioning LTP.
These results in vivo may suggest that posttetanic LTP differs from long-term enhancement after learning by the time course of formation, by the contribution of the EPSP component, and by the extent of glycoprotein synthesis. However, the coincidence of learning ability, of the extent of postconditioning synaptic changes, and of posttetanic LTP may indicate at least a common cellular mechanism or suggests that monosynaptic posttetanic LTP is only a component of the more complex phenomenon of postconditioning LTP, thus only partially or transiently contributing to a long-term memory trace.
Therefore the question arised, if posttetanic LTP represents only one of the regulatory principles mentioned before, thus underlying only a particular memory stage, or would also be based on several subsequent mechanisms and corresponding stages as assumed for the storage of memory traces.
Investigations on hippocampal slices showed that the application of anisomycin, an inhibitor of protein synthesis, during repeated tetanization of Schaffer inputs to CA 1 neurons did not prevent the initiation of LTP and its maintenance during the following 4 hours, but produced a late complete suppression of potentiation without influencing the non-tetanized controls at this time (Frey et al. 1987). This time course corresponds to that of the amnesic effect of anisomycin in vivo. If polymyxin B, an inhibitor of protein kinase C, was applied in a similar manner, posttetanic LTP can also be produced, but the inhibition of potentiation developed already during the

first hour after tetanization, reaching control values
already in the second hour (Reymann et al. 1987).
These results would support the assumption that post-
tetanic LTP
- seems not to be based on a single neuronal mechanism,
- is produced and further maintained with the aid of
  several subsequent processes
Therefore posttetanic LTP during the first hour is not
identical with LTP at later times with regard to the underlying mechanisms, corresponding properties and possibilities to influence physiologically or experimentally
this phenomenon.
From own and other results, we would like to propose that
posttetanic LTP exhibits at least a Ca^{++}/calmodulin-de-
pendent, a protein kinase C-dependent, and an anisomycin-
sensitive stage, shifting from presynaptic to postsynaptic localizations without induction of increased glycoprotein synthesis for a permanent consolidation of synaptic enhancement.

References:

Jork, R., Grecksch, G. and Matthies, H.,(1986), Pharmacol.
Biochem. Behav. 25, 1137-1144

Matthies, H., (1972), Pharmacol. i Toxicol., 35, 259-265

Matthies, H., (1974), Life Sciences, 15, 2017-2031

Matthies, H., (1982), in: Neuronal Plasticity and
Memory Formation, C.A. Marsan and H. Matthies (eds.),
Raven Press New York, pp. 1-15

Matthies, H., Rüthrich, H., Ott, T., Matthies, H.-K.,
and Matthies, R., (1986), Physiol. Behav. 36, 811-821

Pohle, W., Acosta, L., Rüthrich, H., Krug, M. and H.
Matthies, H., (1987), Brain Research, in press

Reymann, K., Frey, U. and Matthies, H., (1987) in this
volume

Frey, U., Krug, M., Reymann, K. and Matthies, H., (1987)
submitted.

Inhibitors of Protein Synthesis, but not mRNA Synthesis, Promote Decay of Long-Term Potentiation in Rat Dentate Gyrus

S. Otani, G. V. Goddard, C. J. Marshall, W. P. Tate, and W. C. Abraham

Department of Psychology and the Neuroscience Center, and Department of Biochemistry, University of Otago, P.O. Box 56, Dunedin, New Zealand

Intraventricular injection of the protein synthesis inhibitor anisomycin for 1 hour just prior to perforant path tetanisation caused LTP of the EPSP in rat dentate gyrus to decay more rapidly over a 3 hour period than controls. Other potent synthesis inhibitors had more moderate effects on LTP decay. The development of LTP was somewhat reduced in all drug conditions. The mRNA synthesis inhibitor, actinomycin D, did not affect either LTP development or its decay. These results suggest that LTP requires new synthesis of proteins, but not mRNAs, for its full development and maintenance.

Morphological (1,2) and biochemical (3) studies have suggested that the mechanisms underlying long-term potentiation (LTP) might involve protein synthesis. This is an attractive hypothesis since 1) the duration of LTP might be longer than the half-lives of certain critical molecules and 2) LTP may be involved in normal information storage which is also considered to involve protein synthesis (e.g. 4). Using inhibitors of protein synthesis, several laboratories have suggested that the occurrence (5,6) or maintenance (7) of LTP is dependent on the degree of protein synthesis at the time of tetanisation. We have examined this question further by testing the effects of several protein synthesis inhibitors (anisomycin, emetine, cycloheximide and puromycin) as well as an inhibitor of mRNA synthesis, actinomycin D, on LTP.

Male albino Sprague-Dawley rats weighing 350-600 g were anesthetized with urethane (1.5g/kg, i.p.). A monopolar recording electrode was unilaterally implanted into the dentate hilus; a stimulating electrode was implanted into the ipsilateral perforant pathway. A 30 gauge stainless steel cannulae implanted into the ipsilateral lateral ventricle was used for drug injection. 0.03 Hz test pulses were delivered throughout the experiment. During the first 60 min period a drug or saline vehicle was injected by 2 µl every 5 min, 12 times. Drug concentrations were: anisomycin 10 µg/µl, emetine, cycloheximide and puromycin 20 µg/µl, and actinomycin D 5 µg/µl. At the end of this drug injection period, LTP was induced by 10 sets of conditioning trains of 20 ms

H.L. Haas G. Buzsàki (Eds.)
Synaptic Plasticity in the Hippocampus
© Springer-Verlag Berlin Heidelberg 1988

duration, 400 Hz and 1 sec apart from another, and the decay was followed for a 3 hour period.

All the protein synthesis inhibitors accomplished 80-90% inhibition of protein synthesis (data for puromycin not available) by the first 30 min after the conditioning as compared to saline controls.

Clear LTP of the population EPSP was induced in all the conditions. Statistical analysis showed no differences between saline and actinomycin D groups on any measure, so these two groups were pooled as the control for further analysis. A comparison between groups at 10 min after tetanisation showed less LTP in the four protein synthesis inhibitor conditions, but which was statistically significant only for the emetine group. (Table 1). Decay of LTP was calculated as follows: [(percent increase after 10 min)-(percent increase after 3 hours)/percent increase after 10 min] x 100. The anisomycin group started to show more decay of LTP of the EPSP after about 30 min and nearly a complete return to baseline after 3 hours. Emetine had a similar effect to anisomycin, but was not as potent. Cycloheximide and puromycin effects on the decay of LTP were about half that of anisomycin. Interestingly there was no significant difference in either the occurrence or decay in LTP of the population spike for any group. The various inhibitors were found to exert little effect themselves on the evoked potentials over a 3 hour period when tested on separate animals not receiving tetanisation.

These results indicate that the blockade of protein synthesis in this paradigm causes mild inhibition of LTP development, and can in some circumstances effectively promote its decay. Those proteins necessary for the development of LTP and its maintenance in the first 3 hours seem to be synthesized from already existing mRNA, since the blockade of mRNA synthesis with actinomycin D did not affect LTP.

The reason for the differences between the various drug groups is not clear. We have no evidence indicating that the different inhibitors preferentially inhibit certain types of proteins. It is, however, possible that the time taken to reach a sufficient level and duration of protein synthesis inhibition to affect LTP differs between drugs. Thus the period of synthesis inhibition might have been shorter for drugs such as cycloheximide and puromycin at the time of tetanisation, resulting in only moderate effects on LTP decay (cf.5).

Funded by the New Zealand Medical Research Council.

Table 1. Effects of various inhibitors on LTP development
and decay, and degree of inhibition.

	% increase in EPSP		% decay of EPSP	% protein synthesis inhibition
	10 min	180 min		
Saline	39.6 (n=13)	24.1	38.1	
Actinomycin D	44.6 (n=9)	28.6	35.0	28 (n=4)
Anisomycin	30.4 (n=10)	4.5[+]	92.9[+]	83 (n=5)
Emetine	27.4 (n=7)[+]	8.7[+]	70.2	77 (n=5)
Cycloheximide	34.2 (n=6)	14.5	57.9	91 (n=5)
Puromycin	32.4 (n=6)	18.4	50.3	-

[+]significantly different from combined Saline/Actinomycin
D controls, $p < 0.05$. Newman-Keuls test.

REFERENCES

1.   Fifkova E., Anderson C.L., Young S.J. and van
      Harreveld, A.   Effect of anisomycin on stimulation-
      induced changes in dendritic spines of the dentate
      granule cells. J.Neurocytol. 11(1982), 183-210.

2.   Fifkova E. and van Harreveld A., Long-lasting
      morphological changes in dendritic spines of dentate
      granular cells following stimulation of the
      entorhinal area. J.Neurocytol, 6 (1977), 211-230.

3.   Duffy C., Teyler T.J. and Shashoua V.E. Long-term
      potentiation in the hippocampal slice: evidence for
      stimulated secretion of newly synthesized proteins.
      Science 212 (1981), 1148-1151.

4.   Shashoua V.E., Biochemical changes in the CNS during
      learning, in The neural basis of behavior. Beckman,
      A. (Ed.) Holliswood, N.Y.: Spectrum publications,
      (1982), 139-164.

5.   Deadwyler S.A., Dunwiddie T. and Lynch G. A critical
      level of protein synthesis is required for long-term
      potentiation.   Synapse 1 (1987), 90-95.

6.   Stanton P.K. and Sarvey J.M.   Blockade of long-term
       potentiation in rat hippocampal CA1 region by
       inhibitors of protein synthesis.   J.Neurosci. 4
       (1984), 3080-3088.

7.   Krug M., Lössner B. and Ott T.   Anisomycin blocks the
       late phase of long-term potentiation in the dentate
       gyrus of freely moving rats.   Brain Res. Bull. 13
       (1984), 39-42.

A Multi-Phase Model of Synaptic Long-Term Potentiation in Hippocampal CA1 Neurones: Protein Kinase C Activation and Protein Synthesis Are Required for the Maintenance of the Trace

K. Reymann, U. Frey, and H. Matthies

Institute of Neurobiology and Brain Research, Academy Sciences of GDR,
Leipziger Strasse 44, 3090 Magdeburg, German Democratic Republic

The third messenger protein kinase C (PKC) and the de novo synthesis of proteins are selectively involved in late phases of long-term potentiation (LTP), but not in its initiation. Whereas polymyxin B, an inhibitor of protein kinase C, blocked LTP 1-2 hours after tetanization, anisomycin, an inhibitor of protein synthesis, resulted in a blockade of LTP from 5-6 hours onward.

The extremely long duration of LTP, its associative properties as well as the possible involvement of the hippocampus in certain memory processes have led to the suggestion that LTP-like changes may be an elementary mechanism for intermediate or long-term memory. Despite numerous investigations, the molecular mechanisms underlying LTP are still unclear. In a previous investigation from our laboratory it was shown that the synthesis of new proteins is critically related to the maintenance of LTP. In freely moving animals intrahippocampal administration of the short acting, reversible protein synthesis inhibitor, anisomycin, blocked LTP at the perforant path-dentate gyrus synapse from 3-4 hours onward (Krug et al. 1984). In order to overcome some limitations of this in vivo study and to prove whether LTP is similarly dependent on de novo protein synthesis in another hippocampal fibre system, we decided to reinvestigate this topic at the Schaffer collateral-CA1 synapses in vitro using conventional extracellular electrophysiological techniques. Our previous investigations had demonstrated that in the CA1 subregion of the rat LTP can last for the life span of the hippocampal slice in vitro (10 hours or more, Reymann et al. 1985).

20 μM anisomycin, which blocks 3/H/leucin-incorporation in the slice preparation by more than 85 %, was bath-applied 160 min immediately following three 100 Hz/1 sec trains. The LTP of both the population EPSP and the population spike was depressed from 5-6 hours onwards (FIG.1). During a late interval (>6 hours) we found for

H.L. Haas G. Buzsàki (Eds.)
Synaptic Plasticity in the Hippocampus
© Springer-Verlag Berlin Heidelberg 1988

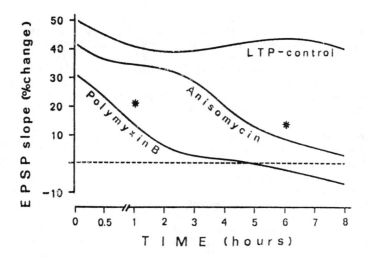

FIG.1: Change in the population EPSP following repeated
tetanization (average percentage change from pre-tetanic
baseline, n=9-12). Control slices exhibited LTP in the
tetanized input which lasted for more than 8 hours.
Perfusion with 20 μM polymyxin B for one hour reduced LTP
persistently and significantly from about one hour
onward(* p<0.05, U-test, two-tailed). Administration of
20 μM anisomycin blocked LTP from 6 hours onward
(p<0.05). In a seperate non-tetanized control input only
small and temporary changes of the response occurred
during drug application. The late heterosynaptic
potentiation of the population spike was, however,
blocked by both drugs (data not shown).

the first time a potentiation of the population spike in
a second, non-tetanized pathway to the same cell
population. This late heterosynaptic potentiation was
also blocked following anisomycin treatment, pointing to
the involvement of postsynaptic processes. These data as
well as preliminary data from our laboratory
demonstrating an enhanced 3/H/ leucin-incorporation
several hours following the induction of LTP (PCHALEK et
al., to be published), substantiate our previous
conclusion that the synthesis of new proteins is
critically related to a late phase of LTP. Thus, as is
the case with memory storage, newly synthetized proteins
are only necessary for the maintenance of the trace, but
not for its initiation.

According to current concepts, intracellular second and
third messengers may mediate metabolic and/or
conformational changes in macromolecules following

receptor activation. The involvement of PKC-mediated processes in mechanisms of LTP was suggested by recent studies which have demonstrated a correlation between PKC-activation and LTP (Akers and Routtenberg 1985, Malenka et al 1986, Lynch and Bliss 1986). However, it was not possible to tell whether there is a causal relationship between the two events. Therefore, we have examined the induction and maintenance of LTP in CA1 hippocampal slices in the presence of a relatively selective PKC-inhibitor. Bath application of 0.1-100 μM polymyxin B sulfate did not influence the occurrence of posttetanic and long-term potentiation usually seen in test responses 1 and 10 minutes after a 100 Hz/1 sec tetanic stimulation of stratum radiatum fibres. However, 20 μM polymyxin B administered during repeated tetanization (3 trains) significantly depressed the increase in population spike amplitude and population EPSP slope from 30-120 min onwards. Immediately after the drug application only non-significant and reversible depressive effects were seen by the same parameters from test responses of the non-tetanized control input. The late heterosynaptic potentiation of the population spike in the control input was also blocked by polymyxin B treatment. Whereas the EPSP-LTP was fully blocked, some significant potentiation of the population spike still remained (50-60 % compared to pre-tetanic baseline), suggesting the independence of PKC of the E/S potentiation. These results provide direct evidence that the PKC-activation is not essential for the initial phase of LTP, but is a necessary condition for a medium and the late, protein synthesis-dependent, phase in this monosynaptic pathway.

In conclusion, these data allow the tentative distinction of 3 seperate phases or partial mechanisms of synaptic long-term potentiation. Neither PKC- nor protein synthesis-dependent processes seem to be involved in the initiation of LTP, i.e. in an early phase (LTP 1). As far as trifluoperazine already blocks early LTP (Finn et al. 1980), a calmodulin-regulated enhancement of presynaptic transmitter release (Lynch and Bliss 1986) may contribute to the genesis of LTP 1. PKC-mediated phosphorylation processes are necessary for an otherwise unidentified medium phase (LTP 2, 1-5 hours). Moreover, PKC-mediated processes as well as a presumably postsynaptic protein synthesis seem to be important for the maintenance of the trace (LTP 3, >6 hours). In the light of these findings, several conclusions on LTP usually resulting from short investigation periods, should be re-examined considering the existence of multiple LTP phases. In addition, it will be of interest to investigate the relationship between the different partial mechanisms.

References:

Akers RF, Routtenberg A (1985), Brain Res 334:147-151
Finn RC, Browning M, Lynch G (1980), Neurosci Lett 19: 103-108
Krug M, Loesssner B, Ott T (1980), Brain Res Bull 13:39-42
Lynch MA, Bliss TVP (1986), Neurosci Lett 65:171-176
Malenka RC, Madison DV, Nicoll RA (1986), Nature 321:175-177
Reymann KG, Malisch R, Schulzeck K, Brödemann R, Ott T, Matthies H. (1985), Brain Res Bull 15:249-255

Modulation of Spike Repolarization in Hippocampal Neurones by Tumor-Promoting Phorbol Esters

J. F. STORM

Department of Neurobiology and Behavior, State University of New York at Stony Brook, Stony Brook, NY 11794, USA

Tumor-promoting phorbol esters (TPEs) are known to enhance synaptic transmitter release. This effect is likely to involve protein kinase C (PKC), which is directly activated by TPEs [3]. In the hippocampus, TPEs induce synaptic enhancement which resembles, and occludes, long-term potentiation (LTP) [8], and LTP has been correlated with translocation of PKC [1]. In Aplysia neurones, another protein kinase (PKA) mediates synaptic enhancement which underlies certain forms of learning [5]. The proposed mechanism in Aplysia is inhibition of a K current, leading to a broadening of the presynaptic action potential, increased Ca influx, and enhanced transmitter release [5]. I am investigating the possibility that a similar mechanism may contribute to synaptic plasticity in the hippocampus.

Intracellular recordings were made from CA1 pyramidal neurons in hippocampal slices from rats (29-35°C). Single action potentials were elicited by injecting brief (1-4ms) depolarizing current pulses. In all cells tested (n=21), the TPEs 4β-phorbol-12,13-diacetate (PDAc) or 4β-phorbol-12,13-dibutyrate (PDBu) (0.3-5μM), broadened the spike [10]. The broadening was only due to slowing of the spike repolarization; the upstroke was unaffected. The effect did not reverse during wash-out for up to 1hr. In contrast to TPEs, 4β-phorbol or 4α-phorbol-12,13-didecanoate, which do not activate PKC [3], were ineffective, suggesting that the effect of PDAc and PDBu was mediated by PKC.

Previous results suggest that at least two active K currents contribute to spike repolarization in CA1 cells [9]: (1) a fast Ca-activated K current (I_C), which can be blocked by 1mM tetraethylammonium (TEA) or Ca-channel blockers [6], and (2) a Ca-independent transient K current (I_A), which is blocked by 0.1mM 4-aminopyridine (4-AP) [4]. Thus, the spike broadening induced by TPEs might be due to inhibition of I_C or I_A. However, neither of these hypotheses were supported by experiments. The spike broadening effect of TPEs did not seem to be due to inhibition of I_C, because: (1) blockade of I_C with TEA, Mn or Cd, did not occlude the effect of subsequent application of TPEs; (2) TPEs applied prior to TEA did not occlude its spike-broadening effect; and (3) the fast after-hyperpolarization, which appears to be mainly due to I_C [9], was not blocked by TPEs. Similarly, I_A did not seem to be involved in the TPE effect, because: (1)

H.L. Haas G. Buzsàki (Eds.)
Synaptic Plasticity in the Hippocampus
© Springer-Verlag Berlin Heidelberg 1988

TPEs still broadened the spike when applied after 0.2mM 4-AP, which blocks I_A; and (2) TPEs did not occlude the spike-broadening effect of 0.1mM 4-AP. Preliminary voltage clamp experiments support the conclusion that I_C or I_A are not reduced by TPEs.

Alternative mechanisms for the spike broadening effect of TPEs, include effects on Na-currents, Ca-currents, the delayed rectifier K-current, the slow Ca-dependent K current, I_{AHP} [6], the voltage-dependent chloride current, $I_{Cl(V)}$ [7], the M-current, the Q-current or the leak current. However, testing of these hypotheses, using current clamp and voltage clamp techniques, has so far failed to yield a conclusive answer. For example, although both I_{AHP} and $I_{Cl(V)}$ are sensitive to TPEs [2,7], they do not appear to be involved in the spike-broadening effect, because: (1) both currents are blocked by 0.2mM Cd [6,7], which did not block the TPE effect.

In conclusion, some phorbol esters broaden the action potential in CA1 hippocampal pyramidal cells. This effect seems to be limited to those phorbol esters which can activate PKC, suggesting that protein phosphorylation is involved, but the ionic mechanism remains to be determined. If a similar PKC-dependent spike broadening occurrs in preynaptic terminals, it may enhance Ca-influx and transmitter release and contribute to synaptic plasticity.[Supported by a Fogarty international fellowship and by NIH Grant NS 18579.]

1 Akers, R.F., Lovinger, D.M., Colley, P.A., Linden, D.J. and Routtenberg, A., Science, 231 (1986) 587-589.

2 Baraban, J.M., Snyder, S.H., and Alger, B.E., Proc.Natl.Acad.Sci. USA,82 (1985) 2538-2542.

3 Castagna, M., Takai, Y., Kaibuchi, K., Sano, K, Kikkawa, U. and Nishizuka, Y., J. biol. Chem. 257 (1982) 7847-7851.

4 Gustafsson, B., Galvan., M., Grafe, P. and Wigström, H.A.,Nature, 299 (1982) 252-254.

5 Klein, M., Shapiro, E. and Kandel, E.R., J. exp. Biol., 89 (1980) 117-157.

6 Lancaster, B. and Adams, P.R., J. Neurophysiol., 55 (1986) 1268-1282.

7 Madison, D.V., Malenka, R.C. and Nicoll, R.A., Nature, 321 (1986) 695-697.

8 Malenka, R.C., Madison, D.V. and Nicoll, R.A., Nature, 321 (1986) 175-177.

9 Storm, J.F., J. Physiol. 385 (1987) 733-759.

10 Storm, J.F., Neurosci. letters 75 (1987) 71-74.

Control of Excitability in Hippocampus

Long-Term Potentiation in Relation to Kindling of the Rat Hippocampus

F. H. Lopes da Silva, W. J. Wadman, W. Kamphuis, B. P. C. Melchers, and J. P. M. Pijn

Department of General Zoology, University of Amsterdam, Kruislaan 320, 1098 SM Amsterdam, The Netherlands

Long-term potentiation (LTP) is a long-lasting facilitation of synaptic transmission which can be put in evidence after a tetanic stimulation of afferent fibers. The kindling process of stimulation, first described by Goddard consists in the application of a series of low intensity tetani to a brain structure such that after a number of repeated applications, after–discharges and epileptic seizures may occur. The question that we address here is how these two phenomena are related, namely whether kindling can be accounted for by an accumulation of LTP.

We examined this question both using in vivo and in vitro techniques. Wistar rats were implanted, under anesthesia, with stimulating and recording electrodes in the hippocampus. The electrodes were aimed at the CA_1 field, with the stimulation electrodes located in the stratum radiatum in order to stimulate the Schaffer collaterals and the recording electrodes placed in the stratum oriens/pyramidale and in the stratum radiatum. In this way, it was possible to obtain optimal recordings of the equivalent dipoles generated by the synaptic activity of the pyramidal cells.

At the initial kindling stages LTP, defined as a potentiation of the top amplitude of the field EPSP and/or of its rising slope, was found but this was ony clear in 5 out of 8 kindled rats. That LTP was not clearly found in all kindled rats may be due to the fact that LTP is not uniformly distributed in space along the pyramidal cells as shown, using current-source-density analysis in vitro and in vivo by Melchers et al. (1986) and by Wadman et al. (1987). In many cases, where LTP was clearly found, this effect tended to saturate at about kindling session 4-6. At later kindling stages another form of potentiation occurred, namely a population spike emerged and increased gradually in amplitude and at a steeper rate than the corresponding field EPSP recorded at the stratum pyramidale. These changes were accompanied by a significant enhancement of Ca^{2+} conductance which was apparent, in vitro, in slices taken from the hippocampus (CA_1) of kindled rats (Wadman et al. 1985). This finding indicates that kindling leads to an enhancement of excitatory aminoacid receptors (e.g. NMDA) mediated Ca^{2+} currents.

Along with these enhanced excitatory phenomena, kindling of the CA_1 field was also characterized by a conspicuous decrease of paired pulse depression (Lopes da Silva 1987, Kamphuis et al. 1987b); this was a continuous process which was apparent from the earliest sessions and reached a saturation level at about sessions 10-12. It indicates a gradual impairment of recurrent inhibition.

H. L. Haas   G. Buzsàki (Eds.)
Synaptic Plasticity in the Hippocampus
© Springer-Verlag Berlin Heidelberg 1988

This phenomenon was related to a long-lasting change in GABA-immunoreactive cell density (Kamphuis et al. 1986, 1987a). The possibility that this change may be related to the intracellular accumulation of Ca^{2+} is under investigation.

Therefore in kindling of CA_1 field the initial LTP effect is accompanied, and probably reinforced, by a disinhibitory process. In this way a positive feedback loop between potentiation and disinhibition takes place.

In conclusion, the kindling process in CA_1 has a LTP component but cannot be reduced to it. It consists of a chain of processes: (i) enhanced excitatory synaptic transmission (LTP); (ii) enhanced Ca^{2+} influx; (iii) impairment of recurrent inhibition; (iv) long-lasting decrease in GABA mediated inhibitory processes. In this way the stability of the underlying neuronal network changes in such a way that even mild stimuli are capable of driving it into oscillatory behaviour. In mathematical terms we may state that the neural network of CA_1 due to the chain of processes characteristic of kindling, is driven into a strange attractor state which, according to preliminary mathematical analysis (Van Neerven, pers. comm.) appears to be of a low dimension.

References

Lopes da Silva, F.H.   Hippocampal kindling: physiological evidence for progressive disinhibition. Advances in Epileptology, 1987, Vol. 16, Ch. 12: 57-62.

Melchers, B.P.C., Lopes da Silva, F.H. and Wadman, W.J.   Long-term potentiation in the hippocampal slice: spatial aspects. In: H. Matthies (Ed.) *Learning and memory: Mechanisms of information storage in the nervous system.* Pergamon Press, Oxford, 1986: 51-60.

Kamphuis, W., Wadman, W.J., Buijs, R.M. and Lopes da Silva, F.H.   Decrease in number of hippocampal gamma-aminobutyric acid (GABA) immunoreactive cells in the rat kindling model of epilepsy. Exp. Brain Res.,1986, 64: 491-495.

Kamphuis, W., Wadman, W.J., Buijs, R.M. and Lopes da Silva, F.H.   The development of changes in hippocampal gamma-aminobutyric acid (GABA) in the rat kindling model of epilepsy: a light microscopic study with GABA-antibodies. Neuroscience, 1987a (in press).

Kamphuis, W., Lopes da Silva, F.H., and Wadman, W.J.   Changes in local evoked potentials in the rat hippocampus (CA_1) during kindling epileptogenesis. Brain Res., 1987b (in press).

Wadman, W.J., Heinemann, U., Konnerth, A. and Neuhaus, S.   Hippocampal slices of kindled rats revealed calcium involvement in epileptogenesis. Exp. Brain Res., 1985, 57: 404-407.

Wadman, W.J., Melchers, B.P.C. and Lopes da Silva, F.H.   Changes in spatial distribution of current sources and sinks during long-term potentiation in the in vitro fascia dentata of the rat. 1987 (submitted for publication).

The Role of M1 and M2 Receptors in Slow Muscarinic Excitation of Hippocampal Neurons

U. Misgeld and W. Müller

Department of Neurophysiology, Max-Planck-Institut für Psychiatrie, Am Klopferspitz 18a, 8033 Planegg-Martinsried, Federal Republic of Germany

Electrical stimulation of presumed septo-hippocampal fibers induced an excitability increase in hippocampal neurons lasting 1-2 min. The excitability increase was due to a membrane depolarization and a diminuition of cell discharge accomodation. Both effects were mimicked by the exogenous application of carbachol (CCh) and blocked by atropine. The depolarization faded with repeated stimulation or during the action of exogenous agonists. The depolarization, but not the diminuition of accomodation, was sensitive to pirenzepine, suggestive of a contributon of M1 and M2 receptors.

The slow "modulatory" effects which can be induced in hippocampal neurons by exogenous cholinergic-muscarinic agonists have been considered relevant to the understanding of memory functions involving hippocampal activity. Some of these slow muscarinic effects can be induced also in slices by the electrical stimulation of presumed septo-hippocampal cholinergic fibers (2,4). In guinea pig hippocampal slices, we investigated the properties of cholinergic-muscarinic effects induced by electrical stimulation or by the exogenous application of CCh. The effects were studied by intracellular recording from CA3 neurons and granule cells in the current clamp or in the single electrode voltage clamp configuration. For the evaluation of CCh effects, some measurements of CCh tissue concentration after bath application were performed using a nominally K-sensitive electrode (5).

Two effects, a membrane depolarization and a reduction of the slow afterhyperpolarization (sAHP) following a train of action potentials, could be elicited in CA3 neurons and granule cells by stimulation with short stimulus trains (0.5-1s, 20-100Hz) applied near the cell layer (2,4). The membrane depolarization, eventually preceeded by a membrane hyperpolarization, could last up to 120s after the stimulus train. In voltage clamp recordings, an apparent slow inward current followed the initial outward current. At a holding potential of -60mV, the inward current was rather small (max. 0.1nA) and associated with a slight conductance decrease. In a potential range of -50 to -40mV, a faster larger inward current component was superimposed, which was

H.L. Haas   G. Buzsàki (Eds.)
Synaptic Plasticity in the Hippocampus
© Springer-Verlag Berlin Heidelberg 1988

associated with a conductance increase. The slow inward current could also be observed at membrane potentials as low as -70 to -80mV if rectifying K-currents were partially blocked by Cs. The membrane depolarization and the inward current, respectively, were enhanced by physostigmine (1uM) and blocked by atropine (1uM) or pirenzepine (0.1-1uM).

A reduction of the sAHP and the outward current that followed a short depolarization from a membrane potential of -60mV could be observed to follow the stimulation of presumed septo-hippocampal fibers without a concomitant depolarization or inward current. As a rule, this was observed in granule cells in the absence of physostigmine. After the application of physostigmine, sAHP and I(AHP), respectively, decreased gradually with time. sAHP and I(AHP) were restored immediately by atropine (1uM), but not by pirenzepine (1-10uM). Exogenous application of CCh (1uM) induced a depolarization and a blockage of the sAHP only if an application mode was chosen so that the CCh concentration in the tissue rose rapidly. With a slow application mode, which resulted in the same tissue concentration, but after a much longer delay, the sAHP was blocked, but the membrane potential remained unchanged.

When the stimulation of septo-hippocampal fibers was repeated at short time intervals (less than 5 min), the resulting inward current was much reduced (Fig.1). Further, the effect of exogenous CCh on the membrane potential faded, even with the CCh concentration in the tissue still increasing. With repetitive applications of CCh at short time intervals, CCh failed to induce further depolarizations, but the sAHP was further reduced. A similar effect was induced by long time exposure to physostigmine. As a result, depolarization induced an inward current, which was sensitive to Ca-antagonists (Ni,Cd) and atropine, but insensitive to pirenzepine. This voltage-dependent inward current underlied the bursting activity of hippocampal neurons, which was observed after repeated CCh applications or in the presence of physostigmine.

As reported elsewhere (1,2), K-currents are the target of muscarinic effects in the hippocampus. Our data indicate that two receptor subtypes, M1 and M2, modulate K-currents of hippocampal neurons. M2 receptors may reduce gK(Ca) and M1 receptors a voltage insensitive gK. Only the M2 receptor mediated effect is continuous. The M1 receptor mediated effect fades rapidly, possibly on account of M1 receptor desensitization(3). Only the M2 receptor mediated effect, therefore, may provide a tonic mechanism for the regulation of cell output frequency.

Supported by a grant to the SFB 220 of the Deutsche Forschungsgemeinschaft.

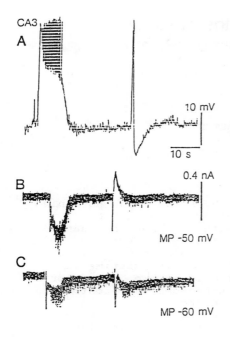

Fig.1:   Fading of the slow EPSP
and the slow EPSC with repeated
stimulation.   Two   consecutive
stimulus   trains   (0.5s,   100Hz)
were   applied   to   the   stratum
oriens of CA3.   The sEPSP and
the sEPSC, respectively, following the second stimulation
are greatly reduced.   A and B
were taken   at the same membrane
potential.

References:

1.   Brown   D.A.,   Gähwiler   B.H.,   Marsh S.J.,   Selyanko
A.A.(1986) Mechanisms of muscarinic excitatory synaptic
transmission in ganglia and brain. TIPS 2, 66-71.
2. Cole,   A.E., Nicoll R.A. (1983) Acetylcholine mediates a
slow synaptic potential in hippocampal pyramidal cells.
Science 221, 1299-1301
3.   Cioffi   C.L.,   El-Fakahany   E.E.   (1986)   Short-term
desensitization of muscarinic cholinergic receptors in
mouse neuroblastoma cells: selective loss of agonist low-
affinity and pirenzepine high-affinity binding sites. J.
Pharmacol.Exp.Therap. 238, 916-923
4.   Müller   W.,   Misgeld   U.   (1986)   Slow   cholinergic
excitation of guinea pig hippocampal neurons is mediated by
two muscarinic receptor subtypes.   Neuroscience Lett. 67,
107-112
5. Müller W., Misgeld U., Heinemann U. (1967) Equilibration
time   course   of   carbachol   in   hippocampal   slices:
significance for muscarinic effects of carbachol. Pflügers
Archiv, 408, R55

Changes in Synaptic Function that Underly Epileptiform Activity in Hippocampal Pyramidal Cells

H. V. WHEAL

Department of Neurophysiology, University of Southampton,
Southampton SO9 3TU, United Kingdom

The role and organisation of the hippocampus not only gives us a unique opportunity to study the synaptic plasticity underlying LTP but also the changes in synaptic function associated with epilepsy. The kainic acid lesioned rat hippocampus has a pattern of cell loss that is similar to that found in temporal lobe epilepsy. In experiments using this chronic animal model of epilepsy we have observed changes in membrane and synaptic mechanisms that contribute to epileptiform bursting activity in the surviving CA1 pyramidal cells. The subject of this paper is to discuss the changes in inhibitory and excitatory synaptic function that underly this behaviour.

Failure of synaptic inhibition.

The intracerebroventricular injection of kainic acid(KA) produces a discrete unilateral lesion of the hippocampal CA3/CA4 area but with very little obvious damage to the CA1 pyramidal cells. However, there was found to be a chronic loss or significant reduction in functional synaptic inhibition in the surviving population of cells in the CA1 region (Lancaster & Wheal, 1984; Cornish & Wheal, 1986). This was expressed at the cellular level by a loss of evoked GABAa -Cl- mediated IPSPs in the pyramidal cells (Ashwood, Lancaster & Wheal, 1986). The loss of inhibition was not associated with changes in postsynaptic responses to GABA iontophoretically applied to either the pyramidal cell soma or dendrites (Ashwood & Wheal, 1986b). This suggests that the mechanism was presynaptic, however it did not appear to be caused by a loss of GABA containing interneurons (Davies, Ashwood, Wheal & Kohler, 1985) or their ability to release GABA when depolarised (unpublished observation). There was also a loss or reduction of the slow IPSP in pyramidal cells, that has been shown to be mediated by a potassium conductance (Ashwood, Lancaster & Wheal, 1986; Newberry & Nicoll, 1984).

NMDA component to the epileptiform EPSP.

Orthodromic activation of the surviving commissural afferents to the CA1 pyramidal cells in the lesioned hippocampus in vitro produces a burst of population spikes, or intracellularly recorded action potentials. We have found

H. L. Haas G. Buzsàki (Eds.)
Synaptic Plasticity in the Hippocampus
© Springer-Verlag Berlin Heidelberg 1988

that a major part of this epileptiform EPSP is contributed
by the activation of N-methyl-D- aspartate(NMDA) receptors
(Ashwood & Wheal, 1986a; 1987). This NMDA-receptor mediated
component of the epileptiform burst was uncovered by the use
of the NMDA antagonist D-2-amino-5-phosphonovalerate(D-APV)
(Watkins & Evans, 1981), and we also confirmed that the
control monosynaptic EPSP evoked by excitatory afferents in
the stratum radiatum was insensitive to NMDA antagonists
(Collingridge et al., 1983; Koerner & Cotman, 1982). Our
observations are an extension of the original evidence that
NMDA antagonists attenuate seizures in vivo (Meldrum et al.
1983) and convulsant- induced epileptiform activity in
hippocampal slices (Herron, Williamson & Collingridge,
1985). However, when GABAa-Cl- mediated inhibition was
reduced with bicuculline so as to produce a similar number
of population spikes to that seen in lesioned slices we
found this acute epileptiform activity to be much less
sensitive to the NMDA antagonist D-APV (Ashwood & Wheal,
1986a). It therefore appears that the NMDA receptor-mediated
event which contributes to the bursting activity in lesioned
slices does not wholly arise as a consequence of the
reduction in the early IPSP.

Discussion.

As yet we have no data to explain the failure of the
early and late synaptic inhibition. One machanism that has
been recently proposed in a kindling model of epilepsy is
that activation of NMDA receptors blocks GABAergic
inhibition (Selzer, Slater & ten Bruggencate, 1987). There
are many similarities in the observations made with this
model and our data on the KA lesioned hippocampus in that
both models show a loss of recurrent and feed-forward IPSPs
as well as the expression of an NMDA receptor-mediated
component to the EPSP. Unfortunately, we have not found any
change in the sensitivity of postsynaptic GABA receptors
associated with the epileptiform activity in our model
(Ashwood & Wheal, 1986b). We would therefore suggest that
the loss of the IPSPs in the KA model might be the
consequence of a loss of excitatory drive to the GABA
containing interneurones or a structural change at the
inhibitory synapses (Ribak, 1985).

There is good evidence for NMDA receptors in the
stratum radiatum of CA1. However, an NMDA-receptor component
to the evoked excitatory response is usually only expressed
in the hippocampal slices when they are exposed to low
extracellular Mg++ (Herron et al., 1985) which removes the
voltage dependent Mg++ block of the channels linked to the
NMDA receptors (Nowak et al., 1984). While the long
duration epileptiform EPSP was recorded in the presence of
Mg++ we have no data that suggests that the amplitude of the
epileptiform EPSP in the soma was sufficient to overcome the
Mg++ block. Of course there may be a much larger
depolarisation at the site of the excitatory synapses on the
apical dendrites of the pyramidal cells. An alternative
mechanism for the expression of an NMDA-receptor component

to the epileptiform EPSP might involve plasticity of the excitatory synapses, similar to the induction of LTP (Wigstrom & Gustafsson, 1984).

Conclusion.

We have described changes in both inhibitory and excitatory synaptic function that contribute to the epileptiform activity in a chronic model of epilepsy. It is tempting to suggest that loss of synaptic inhibition leads to the expression of an NMDA-receptor mediated component to the epileptiform EPSP, however loss of just the early bicuculline sensitive IPSP may not be enough to uncover this mechanism. The additional loss of the late K+ mediated IPSP might also be required. What ever the postulated mechanism is for the induction of the NMDA component of epileptiform activity, it would be difficult not to include a potentiating role for glycine (Johnson & Ascher, 1987), especially as high levels of glycine have been found to be associated with epileptogenic foci in the human brain (Van Gelder, Sherwin & Rasmussen, 1977).

This work was supported by grants from the MRC and the Wellcome Trust. H.V.W. is a Wellcome Senior Lecturer.

References.

Ashwood TJ, Wheal HV (1986a) Extracellular studies on the role of N-methyl-D-aspartate receptors in epileptiform activity recorded from the kainic acid lesioned hippocampus. Neurosci Lett 67: 147-152.
Ashwood TJ, Wheal HV (1986b) Loss of inhibition in the CA1 region of the kainic acid lesioned hippocampus is not associated with changes in the postsynaptic responses to GABA. Brain Res 367: 390-394.
Ashwood TJ, Lancaster B, Wheal HV (1986) Intracellular electrophysiology of CA1 pyramidal neurones in slices of the kainic acid lesioned hippocampus of the rat. Exp Brain Res 62: 189-198
Ashwood TJ, Wheal HV (1987) The expression of an NMDA-receptor mediated component during epileptiform synaptic activity in the hippocampus. Brit. J. Pharm (In Press).
Collingridge GL, Kehl SJ, McLennan H (1983) Excitatory amino in synaptic transmission in the Schaffer collateral-commissural pathway of the rat hippo-campus. J Physiol 334: 33-46.
Cornish SM, Wheal HV (1986) The long term failure of inhibition in the chronic kainic acid model of temporal lobe epilepsy. Neurosci Lett Suppl 24: S36.

Davies SW, Ashwood TJ, Wheal HV, Kohler C (1985)
    Glutamate decarboxylase(GAD) and GAD immuno-
    reactivity(GDI) in the CA1 region of the kainic
    acid lesioned rat hippocampus. Neurosci Lett
    Suppl 21: S43.

Herron CE, Williamson R, Collingridge GL (1985) A
    selective N-methyl-D-aspartate antagonist
    depresses epileptiform activity in rat hippo-
    campal slices. Neurosci Lett 61: 225-260.

Johnson JW, Ascher P (1987) Glycine potentiates the
    NMDA response in cultured mouse brain neurones.
    Nature 325: 529-531.

Koerner JF, Cotman CW (1982) Response of Schaffer
    collateral CA1 pyramidal cell synapses of the
    hippocampus to analogues of acidic amino acids.
    Brain Res 251: 105-115.

Lancaster B, Wheal HV (1984) Chronic failure of
    inhibition in the CA1 area of the hippocampus
    following kainic acid lesions of the CA3/4 area.
    Brain Res 295: 317-324.

Meldrum BS, Croucher MJ, Badman G, Collins JF (1983)
    Antiepileptic action of excitatory amino acid
    antagonists in the photosensitive baboon Papio
    papis. Neurosci Lett 39: 101-104.

Newberry NR, Nicoll RA (1984) A bicuculline-resistant
    inhibitory post-synaptic potential in rat hippo-
    campal pyramidal cells in vitro. J Physiol
    348: 239-254.

Nowak L., Bregestovski P, Ascher P, Herbet A,
    Prochiantz A (1984) Magnesium gates glutamate-
    activated channels in mouse central neurones.
    Nature 307: 462-465.

Ribak CE (1985) Axon terminals of GABAergic chandilier
    cells are lost at epileptic foci. Brain Res
    326: 251-260.

Stelzer A, Slater NT, ten Bruggencate G (1987)
    Activation of NMDA receptors blocks GABAergic
    inhibition in an in vitro model of epilepsy.
    Nature 326: 698-701.

Van Gelder NM, Sherwin AL, Rasmussen T (1977) Amino
    acid content of epileptogenic human brain:
    Focal versus surrounding regions. Brain Res
    40: 385-397.

Watkins JC, Evans RH (1981) Excitatory amino acid
    transmitters. Ann Rev Pharm Toxicol 21: 165-204.

Wigstrom H, Gustafsson B (1984) A possible correlate of
    the postsynaptic condition for long-lasting
    potentiation in the guinea pig hippocampus in
    vitro. Neurosci Lett 44: 327-332.

Calcium and Long-Term Potentiation in the Rat Hippocampus In Vitro

R. ANWYL, D. MULKEEN, and M. ROWAN[1]

Department of Physiology and Pharmacology[1] Trinity College, Dublin 2, Ireland

Abstract

The magnitude of LTP of the epsp in the rat hippocampus was found to be highly dependent on external Ca, with LTP increasing from 5% in 0.8 mM Ca to 65% in 2.5 mM Ca. The power relationship of 2.1 between the amplitude of the low frequency epsp and the external Ca was not altered by LTP production. The Ca agonist BAY K8644 enhanced LTP, while verapamil, although not affecting the control LTP, did block the enhanced LTP produced by BAY K8644

External Ca has previously been found to be very important in the production of LTP in the hippocampus. Tetanic stimulation in the absence of Ca failed to produce LTP, and decreasing external Ca or increasing external Mg was found to decrease the probability of LTP production (1,2).

In the present studies, we have investigated several aspects of the involvement of Ca in LTP production. These include quantitative studies on the dependency of LTP on extracellular Ca, possible changes in Ca cooperativity of transmitter release following inducement of LTP, and the effects of the Ca agonist BAY K8644 on LTP.

Transverse slices of the rat hippocampus were prepared according to standard methods, and extracellular field recordings of epsp's obtained from the stratum radiatum of CA1 in response to stimulation of the Schaffer collateral-commissural pathway. LTP was studied by giving test pulses which evoked 300 uV amplitude epsp's at 0.02 Hz, and then eliciting a tetanus (20 trains at 0.5 Hz, 9 stimuli per train at 200 Hz) with an epsp amplitude of 900 uV. LTP was expressed as the % increase of the test epsp at 20 min following the tetanus.

Effect of Ca on LTP Amplitude

The magnitude of LTP evoked by a train of stimuli was studied in external Ca concentrations between 0.7 - 2.5 mM. LTP was highly dependent on the Ca concentration of the perfusate, with LTP increasing as the Ca concentration was raised. A plot of LTP against the external Ca concentration showed a very steep relationship between Ca concentrations of 0.8 - 1.0 mM Ca. Thus LTP measured 5 ± 2%, n = 5 in 0.8mM Ca, and 38 ± 7%, n = 5 in 1.0mM Ca (mean $\pm$ SEM). The increase in LTP was much less steep between 1.0 - 2.0mM Ca (LTP in 2mM Ca was 65 ± 4%, n = 6). LTP declined to 38 ± 6%, n = 5 in 2.5mM Ca. The very steep increase in LTP between Ca concentrations of 0.7 - 1.0 mM may be caused by co-

H. L. Haas G. Buzsàki (Eds.)
Synaptic Plasticity in the Hippocampus
© Springer-Verlag Berlin Heidelberg 1988

operativity of Ca action at the molecular complex responsible
for LTP initiation.

Effect of LTP on Ca Cooperativity of Transmitter Release

The amplitude of the epsp evoked at low frequency (0.02Hz)
increased as the external Ca concentration was raised. In these
experiments, the epsp amplitude in 2mM Ca was adjusted to 300 uV,
and the Ca concentration either increased or decreased. The
change in epsp amplitude was expressed as the percentage change to
the amplitude in 2mM Ca. A plot of the relationship between the
epsp amplitude and the external Ca concentration on double logar-
ithmic cooordinates showed that the slope of the regression line
was 2.1 between Ca concentrations of 0.8 - 1.0 mM, and 1.3 between
1.0 - 1.5mM Ca.

Following LTP production in 2 mM Ca, the slope of the relationship
between the epsp emplitude and LTP was not significantly changed,
signifying that LTP does not produce any change in the Ca cooperat·
ivity of transmitter release.

The Ca channel against BAY K8644 was found to potentiate LTP. Thus
in 15 uM BAY K8644, with 0.5% ethanol as vehicle, LTP was 57 $\pm$ 4%,
n=9 (mean $\pm$ SEM). This was a significant increase over the ethanol
control (LTP = 15 $\pm$ 4%, n=9) which itself was a significant
decrease compared with the control in the absence of ethanol (LTP =
43 $\pm$ 10%, n=10). The organic Ca channel antagonist verapamil
inhibited the potentiating effects of BAY K8644, but did not block
the control LTP. When 10 uM verapamil was applied solely with 0.5%
ethanol, LTP measured 27 $\pm$ 8%, n=5, a value not significantly
different from the vehicle control. Moreover, in 10 uM verapamil
applied together with BAY K8644 and ethanol, LTP measured 28 $\pm$ 7%
n=5, which was also not significantly different from the vehicle
control.

The enhancement of LTP by BAY K8644 may demonstrate that Ca entry
through voltage dependent Ca channels initiates part of the LTP,
since BAY K8644 acts by prolonging opening of voltage dependent Ca
channels (3). Alternatively, BAY K8644 may have another site of
action, such as that which increased spontaneous transmitter
release even in the absence of Ca at the neuromuscular junction (4)

References:

1.   Wigstrom, H., Swan, J.W. and Anderson, P.
      Acta Physiol Scand. 105, 126-128 (1979)

2.   Dunwiddie, T.V. & Lynch, G. Brain Res 169, 103-110 (1979)

3.   Nowycky, M.C. Fox, A.P. & Tsien, R.R. Proc. Nath Acad Sci
      USA 82, 2178-2182 (1985)

4.   O'Leary, S.M & Atchinson, W.D. Soc. Neurosci 1987, 823

Memory-Affecting Drugs and Hippocampal Synaptic Plasticity

M. W. Brown, I. P. Riches, N. J. Cairns, and J. E. Smithson

Department of Anatomy, University of Bristol, Bristol, BS8 1TD, United Kingdom

The effects on paired-pulse and long-term potentiation of drugs which may affect memory have been investigated using rat hippocampal slices. Vincamine and lorazepam blocked long-term potentiation of the field EPSP and population spike recorded in subfield CA1. Vincamine reduced paired-pulse potentiation of the field EPSP. Lorazepam reduced, while vasopressin and pramiracetam increased the excitability of the population spike. These changes resulted in a variety of effects on paired-pulse potentiation of the population spike.

The effects upon hippocampal potentiation of various drugs which may affect performance in memory tests have been investigated. Vasopressin has been claimed (De Wied, 1980) to facilitate the performance of tasks requiring avoidance learning. Both vincamine (Giurgea et al. 1981), an alkaloid, and pramiracetam (Butler, et al. 1984), a derivative of piracetam, have been claimed to enhance memory performance of elderly subjects with poor memories. Lorazepam, a benzodiazepine, has been shown to impair acquisition in humans (Brown et al. 1983).

Hippocampal slices (400 μm) were prepared from male Wistar rats and maintained in oxygenated artificial CSF at $36 \pm 1°C$. Electrical pulses of varying intensity and frequency were applied to the stratum radiatum of subfield CA3. Field EPSPs and population spikes were recorded extracellularly from strata radiatum and pyramidale of subfield CA1. Pairs of pulses separated by times from 10ms to 1s were delivered every 5s, to induce paired-pulse potentiation. Trains of pulses (8 trains of 8 pulses at 400 Hz, at one train per 5s) were used to induce long-term potentiation. A single slice from each rat was used in studies of paired-pulse potentiation, a pair of slices from each rat in long-term potentiation experiments. The effects of drugs were investigated by introducing them into the perfusion medium, >20 min being allowed for washing in and washing out. The significance of quoted effects was established by analyses of variance performed upon logarithmically transformed data.

Excitability: The magnitude of the potential evoked by a single pulse in the presence of a drug was compared to control values. None of the drugs significantly affected the slope of the field EPSP. The mean amplitude of the population spike was significantly increased by 20% by vasopressin (2μM; n=7 rats) and by 20% by pramiracetam (40μM; n=6). Vincamine (100μM; n=7) had no effect, while lorazepam (1μM; n=5)

H. L. Haas G. Buzsàki (Eds.)
Synaptic Plasticity in the Hippocampus
© Springer-Verlag Berlin Heidelberg 1988

significantly reduced the mean amplitude of the population spike by 45%. The lorazepam effect was dose-dependent over the range 10^{-9} to 10^{-5} M and lasted for >30 min after washout.

Paired-pulse potentiation (PPP): Vincamine (100μM; n=7) was the only drug significantly to affect PPP of the field EPSP. It produced a significant reduction of PPP for interpulse intervals of 15-100ms and currents of 150-250% of the threshold for production of the population spike. This reduction was due to a decrease in the amplitude of the field EPSP evoked by the second pulse in the presence of vincamine.

PPP of the population spike was reduced in the presence of vasopressin (2μM; n=7) at intervals of 10-400ms and currents of 200-275% of threshold. The reduction in PPP was due to the vasopressin-induced increase in amplitude of the population spike in response to the first pulse, while the amplitude of the population spike to the second pulse was unchanged by the drug.

Pramiracetam (40μM, n=6) had no net effect on PPP since both the first and second population spikes underwent proportionate increases in size in the presence of the drug.

PPP was increased by lorazepam (15μM; n=8) at short (15-200ms) but not long (250-1000ms) interpulse intervals for a range of currents (150-400% of threshold). This increase was secondary to a reduction of the first, but not the second population spike at intervals $\leqslant$ 150ms. However, if the current was increased so that the first population spike in the presence of lorazepam (1μM; n=6) was no longer reduced compared to control values, a decrease in PPP at short (10-50ms) interspike intervals was seen. This decrease was due to a reduction in the second population spike (probably as a result of enhanced GABA-ergic recurrent inhibition).

Long-term potentiation (LTP): Compared to control values, vincamine (100μM; n=4) and lorazepam (1μM, n=6) both significantly reduced LTP of the field EPSP and of the population spike measured >10 min after high frequency stimulation. Indeed, the drugs could be said to have blocked LTP since the residual potentiation in each case did not differ significantly from zero. Pramiracetam (40μM) was without effect on LTP; the effect of vasopressin was not investigated.

Summary Table

Drug	Excitability	Potentiation	
		PPP	LTP
Vincamine	−	EPSP↓	EPSP↓
Pramiracetam	PS1↑,PS2↑	−	−
Vasopressin	PS1↑	PS↓	
Lorazepam	PS1↓,PS2(↓)	PS↑↓	EPSP↓

Long-term potentiation was blocked by both vincamine (see also Olpe et al. 1982a) and lorazepam. If LTP is related to memory, the effect of vincamine is counter to its proposed memory-enhancing properties, while that of lorazepam is consistent with its amnesic action. Diazepam, a benzodiazepine which is related to lorazepam and is also a secondary amine, has been shown to be an N-methyl-D-aspartate (NMDA) antagonist (Evans et al. 1977). Activation of NMDA receptors is necessary for the production of LTP in the system studied (Collingridge et al. 1983). A number of secondary and tertiary amines have been found to antagonise NMDA (Blake et al. 1987). Note that vincamine is also a tertiary amine which blocks LTP. However, pramiracetam has both secondary and tertiary amine groups but had no effect on LTP.

Excitability and paired-pulse potentiation were affected by the various drugs in different ways. Again, the effects were not consistently correlated with their putative mnemonic properties. Vincamine reduced PPP of the field EPSP, once more an effect not to be expected of a supposedly memory-enhancing agent. All other effects were on the population spike rather than the field EPSP, i.e. the locus of change was post-synaptic. Pramiracetam increased excitability, in keeping with its suggested memory-enhancing role, but did not alter potentiation (PPP or LTP). This effect is similar to that of 1mM piracetam (Olpe et al. 1982b). Vasopressin increased excitability of the CA1 pyramidal cells in response to the first pulse, either by action on interneurones and/or by changes in membrane properties of the CA1 pyramidal cells; it correspondingly reduced PPP. The relation of such changes to any mnemonic effects of vasopressin are unclear. Lorazepam decreased the population spike, its more complex effects on PPP probably being due to the interaction between the decrease in pyramidal cell excitability and the enhanced action of GABA-ergic mechanisms within local circuits. However, its amnesic actions may more probably result from its effects on LTP either within the hippocampus or elsewhere.

References

Blake, J.F. Brown, M.W., Al-Ani, N., Coan, E.J. and Collingridge, G.L. (1987) Mecamylamine blocks responses to NMDA and a component of synaptic transmission in rat hippocampal slices. Proceedings of this meeting.
Brown, J., Brown, M.W. and Bowes, J.B. (1983) Effects of lorazepam on rate of forgetting, on retrieval from semantic memory and on manual dexterity. Neuropsychologia, 21, 501-512.
Butler, D.E., Nordin, I.C., L'Italien, Y.J., Zweisler, L., Doschel, P.H. and Marriott, J.G. (1984). Amnesia-reversal activity of N-[(disubstituted -amino) alkyl] - 2 - oxo - 1 - pyrrolidineacetamides, including pramiracetam. J. of Med. Chem., 27, 684-691.
Collingridge, G.L., Kehl, S.J., McLennan, H. (1983). Excitatory amino acids in synaptic transmission in the Schaffer collateral-commissural pathway of the rat hippocampus. J. Physiol. (Lond.), 334, 33-46.
De Wied, D. (1980). Behavioural actions of neurohypophysial peptides. Proc. R. Soc. (Lond.)B 210, 183-195.

Evans, R.H., Francis, A.A., Watkins, J.C. (1977). Differential antagonism by chlorpromazine and diazepam of frog motoneurone depolarization induced by glutamate-related amino acids. Eur. J. Pharmacol., 44, 325-330.

Giurgea, C., Greindl, G. and Preat, S. (1981). Experimental behavioural pharmacology of gerontopsychopharmacological agents. In F. Hoffmeister (Ed.), Psychotropic Agents, Part II, Springer-Verlag, Berlin.

Olpe, H.R., Barrionuevo, G. and Lynch, G. (1982a). Vincamine: a psychogeriatric agent blocking synaptic potentiation in the hippocampus. Life Sci., 31, 1947-1953.

Olpe, H.R. and Lynch, G. (1982b). The action of piracetam on the electrical activity of the hippocampal slice preparation: a field potential analysis. Eur. J. Pharmacol., 80, 415-419.

This work was supported by the MRC.

Optical Monitoring of Electrical Activity in Hippocampal Slices Using a Voltage Sensitive Dye (RH155)

U. KUHNT

Max-Planck-Institut für Biophysikalische Chemie, 3400 Göttingen,
Federal Republic of Germany

Summary: Absorption measurements were performed in CA1 of hippocampal slices using the voltage sensitive dye RH155. Absorption signals were recorded by a 10x10 photodiode array, and the distribution of optical signals was analyzed. Presynaptic components were pharmacologically separated. No influence of the dye was found on the induction and maintenance of LTP and on double pulse facilitation.

Optical recording techniques to monitor membrane potential in neurones have created increasing interest in various fields of neurobiology (for ref. see part 2 in [1]). First reports of successfully monitoring absorption signals with voltage-sensitive probes in mammalian brain slices have appeared since 1980 [3,4,8]. The various dyes, which have so far been tested, all have disadvantages. A good combination of features such as photodynamic damage, bleaching, binding, pharmacologic action, linear change of absorption with voltage and fast changes to voltage steps were scarcely found. It will be shown that RH155, which belongs to the pyrazo-oxonol family (originally synthesized by R. Hildesheim [2]), fulfills most requirements for a good indicator of voltage changes in mammalian brain slices.

Transverse hippocampal slices (350 μm thick) were placed in a recording chamber mounted on an inverted microscope. The chamber was perfused by a standard solution [9]. Stimulating electrodes were placed in the apical dendritic area and occasionally in the str. oriens. A recording electrode monitored continuously the extracellular activity. Slices were stained with RH155 (NK3041 [10]) (1 mg/ml) for 12 min. Transmission mode was used to monitor absorption changes. A 25x or a 40x objective formed an image on the 10x10 photodiode array which was placed in the real image plane of the inverted microscope. With these objectives an area of $(50\mu m)^2$ or $(35\mu m)^2$ of tissue is projected on a single photodiode. Amplification and data recording were similar as described earlier [3], but a sample and hold circuit was used which allows DC-recording. Amplifier outputs were multiplexed and digitized (maximal time resolution 0.3 ms for 100 channels).

Stimulation of unstained slices gives rise to slow changes in absorption, seen at all wavelengths. The intrinsic signal (or light scatter) begins at the same time as the electrical activity and may be caused by biochemical changes. The ab-

H. L. Haas   G. Buzsàki (Eds.)
Synaptic Plasticity in the Hippocampus
© Springer-Verlag Berlin Heidelberg 1988

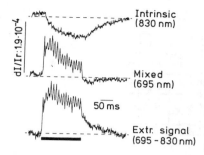

Intrinsic (830 nm)

dI/Ir·1·9·10⁻⁴

Mixed (695 nm)

50 ms

Extr. signal (695 - 830 nm)

Fig. 1: Separation of intrinsic and extrinsic signals: Intrinsic (top row, measured at 830 nm), mixed (middle, 695 nm) and calculated extrinsic signal (bottom). The records are averaged responses (N=2) to a stimulus train (100 Hz/180 ms, marked by a black bar at bottom). Area: (35 µm)². Light increase downwards. Calibration of time and fractional change as indicated.

sorbance change monitored after staining consists of the mixed intrinsic and extrinsic (caused by the dye) signals. To obtain the unaffected extrinsic signal, the intrinsic signal must be subtracted. Since RH155 does not absorb at wavelengths around 830 nm, this wavelength is used to record exclusively intrinsic signals. Maximal absorption changes were recorded at ~700 nm. Fig. 1 demonstrates the distortion of the extrinsic signal caused by the intrinsic signal. The upper record shows the response to a stimulus train of a stained slice at 830 nm. The middle record shows the mixed signal, measured at 695 nm and the lower record shows the result of the subtraction. Interpretation based on mixed signals are misleading, it is therefore essential to record absorption changes under both conditions.

The responses to double pulse stimulation begin with a transient signal. The spatial location of the maximum depends on the position of the stim. el. in the apical dendrites. The amplitude decays proximally and distally from the maximum, maximal amplitude and decay depend on stimulus strength. These signals persist in Ca-free solution, at high Mg-concentrations, and after addition of Cd. Application of TTX abolishes the transient signals, which presumably reflect presynaptic fibre activity. The presynaptic signal is followed by a slow decrease in absorption. The maximum is mostly seen at or near the location with the highest presynaptic signal. At higher stimulus strengths a transient absorption decrease develops, this is most strongly expressed at the level of the pyramidal cell somata. Both components disappear if Ca is omitted or if Cd is added. Furthermore glutamyldiethylester (GDEE) strongly depresses this response [7]. The presynaptic responses to a double stimulus are very similar, but the slow response to the second stimulus is strongly facilitated. The slow responses reflect the summed depolarization of the evoked EPSPs. The transient signal which originates in the pyramidal cell layer decays with distance from the soma, it might be caused by action potentials. Fig. 2a shows absorption changes in response to a double stimulus along the apical dendritic axis. Presynaptic signals (I, I') decrease in amplitude from record 8 which is about 300-400 µm away from the somata in the direction of the cell layer (line 1-2). The evoked action potential (II, II') is largest in the cell layer (1-2) and decreases distally. With low stimulus intensities the separation of pre- and postsynaptic components is difficult and Ca-free solutions

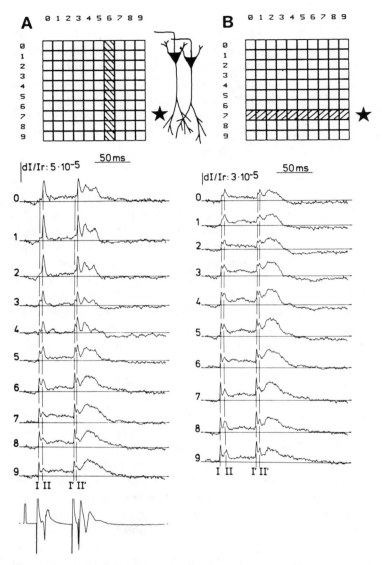

Fig. 2: Distribution of optical signals: Corrected optical signals (average, N=10) to double pulse stimulation (separation 50 ms). Each record represents activity of (50 μm)² tissue area. Orientation of tissue and diode array are shown in the top diagrams. Pyramidal cell layer is located approximately at line 1 and 2. Calibr. (time and fractional change) as indicated. Light increase downwards. I and I' indicate presynaptic, II and II' postsynaptic activity to the first and second stimulus, respectively. The numbers on the records correspond to the position of the diode, A: diode 0-9 of column 6, B: diode 0-9 of line 7. At the bottom of A is shown the extracellular response, recorded in the pyramidal cell layer. The asterisk shows the approximate position of stim. electrode.

or pharmacological agents are necessary to uncover the presynaptic component. With increasing distance from the stimulating electrode, the amplitude of the presynaptic potential and the width of the activated bundle along the apical dendrites diminishes. Over a distance of about 500 μm the amplitude decreases by 50-70 %. The postsynaptic response also decreases with distance. The maximal response is often spatially separated from the maximal presynaptic response. Such a situation is shown in Fig. 2b.

Short trains of stimuli induce large absorption signals which exceed the amplitude of control responses at the same stimulus strength. Fig. 1 shows an average of 2 responses to a train of stimuli. The transient signals on top of the broad plateau of the corrected signal (bottom record) represent action potentials, the largest amplitudes of these transients are regularly seen at and near the pyramidal cell layer. Following high frequency stimulation, control responses were facilitated. This increase of response amplitudes is stable for at least 3 h. Tetanic stimulation during the application of NMDA-receptor antagonists does not induce longlasting increases of control responses [7].

The oxonol dye RH155, commercially available as NK3041 [10] proved to be a useful voltage sensitive probe for absorption measurements in guinea pig brain slices. The washout and bleaching of bound dye is low and allows exposure times up to 10 min after staining. Pharmacological effects of the dye on the electrical response are not evident; double pulse facilitation and the induction and maintenance of long-term potentiation is not influenced. It is not yet clear if and how much the dye binds to membranes of glial elements and how strongly the recorded signals are influenced by glial responses. Compared with other findings [5,6] in other preparations, the activity of glial cells seems to add less to the absorption signal in guinea pig hippocampal slices. Maximal changes in absorbance were $\Delta I/I = \sim 5 \cdot 10^{-4}$. Stimulation near threshold (as judged from the extracell. rec.) evokes recognizable optical signals, however, averaging is necessary to increase the signal/noise ratio. The final proof that the recorded signal is of exclusively neuronal origin is still elusive; one solution may be to investigate optical signals during intracellular current injections. Our results suggest that the voltage sensitive absorption dye RH155 may be useful for the solution of many problems related to the spatial distribution of voltage changes or related to the correlation of pre- and postsynaptic activity.

References: 1.De Weer P, Salzberg BM (eds.) Optical methods in cell physiology (1986) Wiley-Interscience, New York. 2.Grinvald A, Hildesheim R, Gupta R, Cohen LB (1980) Biol Bull 159:484. 3.Grinvald A, Manker A, Segal M (1982) J Physiol 333:269-291. 4.Grinvald A, Ross WN, Farber I, Saya D, Zutray A, Hildesheim R, Kuhnt U, Segal M, Kimhi Y (1980) In: Littauer (ed) Neurotransmitters and their receptors. Wiley, New York, pp 531-546. 5.Konnerth A, Obaid AL, Salzberg BM. J Physiol (in press). 6.Konnerth A, Orkand RK (1986) Neurosci

Lett 66:49-54. 7.Kuhnt U (1986) Neurosci Lett Suppl 26:S535. 8.Kuhnt U, Grinvald A (1981) Pflügers Arch Suppl 394:R45. 9.Kuhnt U, Mihaly A, Joo F (1983) Brain Res 279:19-30. 10.RH155 is now commercially available as NK3041 from Nippon Kankoh-Shikiso Kenkyusho Co, Ltd., 2-3, Shimoishii 1-chome, Okayama 700, Japan.

Arecoline Induces Theta Rhythm, Reduces Pyramidal Cell Excitability and Moderately Impairs LTP In Vivo

H. R. Olpe, H. Jutzeler, E. Kueng, P. Campiche, K. Klebs, and M. F. Pozza

Biology Research Laboratories, Pharmaceuticals Division, Ciba-Geigy Ltd., 4002 Basle, Switzerland

Abstract:

In the urethane anaesthetized rat arecoline, oxotremorine and physostigmine administered intravenously induce theta activity and reduce the population spike amplitude of CA1 pyramidal neurons evoked by stimulation of the ipsilateral Schaffer commissural fibres. Arecoline dose-dependently and reversibly reduces the epsp. All effects are blocked by atropine. Arecoline moderately attenuates LTP in CA1. Atropine had no effect. These findings indicate that cholinomimetics only partly mimic the action of endogenous acetylcholine.

The hippocampal cholinergic fibres deriving from the medial septum are of particular interest in the context of the Alzheimer's disease because degeneration of forebrain cholinergic neurons are believed to contribute towards the aetiopathology of dementia. It is thought that the administration of cholinomimetics might restore cholinergic function in the brain. The present study adresses the question whether exogenously applied cholinomimetic drugs mimic the action of endogenous acetylcholine in the hippocampus and how they affect LTP induced in this structure.
For this purpose we investigated the actions of intravenously administered cholinergic agonists, of the cholinesterase blocker physostigmine and of atropine on two parameters of hippocampal activity that are thought to be affected by the cholinergic septal input, viz. theta-wave activity and the excitability of pyramidal cells. In a separate series of experiments the effect of systemically applied arecoline or atropine on LTP induced in CA1 was investigated. Since acetylcholine is generally thought to activate pyramidal cells via blockade of the M-current, we were expecting to find that cholinomimetics would increase the excitability of pyramidal cells and thereby facilitate LTP.

Experiments were performed on 44 male Sprague-Dawley rats weighing 280-340 g. The animals were anaesthetized with urethane (1200 mg/kg i.p.) and mounted in a stereo-

H. L. Haas   G. Buzsàki (Eds.)
Synaptic Plasticity in the Hippocampus
© Springer-Verlag Berlin Heidelberg 1988

tactic apparatus. All animals were pretreated with 0.3
mg/kg i.v. of methylscopolamine in order to block peripheral muscarinic receptors. Hippocampal theta activity
was recorded monopolarly by means of a concentric bipolar
electrode (diameter 0.3 mm). Spectral analysis was performed with a CF 300 FFT analyzer (Ono Sokki Co.). Blood
pressure was measured routinely. The excitability of
pyramidal cells was assessed by measuring the amplitude
of the population spike in CA1 induced by stimulating the
Schaffer commissural fibre tract. Conventional recording
and averaging techniques were used. In separate experiments the action of arecoline on the dendritic epsp in CA1
was determined. The effect of intravenously administered
arecoline or atropine on LTP was assessed in two separate
series of experiments. In both series LTP was induced by
administering two trains of stimuli to the Schaffer commissural fibres at an interval of 10 minutes. Each train lasted 200 msec, 100 Hz, each pulse lasting 0.1 msec. The voltage was adjusted to evoke a half-maximal population spike
amplitude if applied as a single pulse. In the arecoline
treated rats the first train of stimuli was given 3 min.
following drug administration.

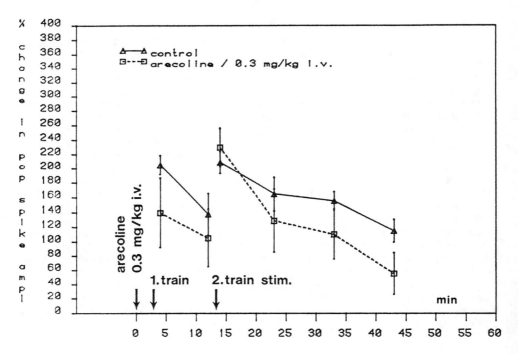

Fig. 1. The depressant effect of arecoline on the induction of LTP in CA1 is depicted. LTP was induced by two
consecutive trains of pulses (n = 7).

Oxotremorine, arecoline and physostigmine evoked theta-wave activity in the hippocampus that was readily blocked by atropine. However, pyramidal cell excitability was reduced dose-dependently by these drugs as indicated by the reduction of the dendritic epsp and the population spike amplitude. Atropine or scopolamine (2 or 5 mg/kg i.v.) almost completely antagonized these effects. These changes were not due to a reduction in blood pressure since it was only minimally affected. Arecoline, at a dose of 0.3 mg/kg i.v. depressed the population spike reversibly and recovery from depression was observed within 10 min. In the experiments in which LTP was induced by two consecutive trains of stimuli arecoline (0.3 mg/kg) impaired the potentiation (PTP) measured 1 min. and LTP measured up to 35 min. later.

The second train of stimuli applied 10 min. after the first one elicited a much larger immediate potentiation measured 1 min. following stimulation. The immediate potentiation was similar to the one recorded in untreated control animals. Interestingly however, this potentiation decayed faster in the arecoline treated than in the untreated animals. In atropine treated rats (n = 7) the immediate potentiation measured 1 min. following the first LTP induction was reduced by 20 % only (Fig. 2).

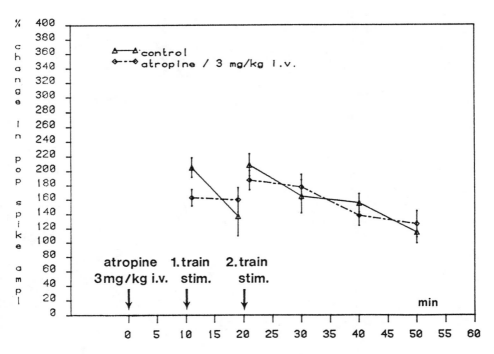

Fig. 2. The effect of atropine on the induction of LTP in CA1 is depicted.

Following the second train of pulses a similar potentiation
of the population spike and a similar time-course of decay
of the potentiation was observed as in control animals.

In conclusion, we found that cholinomimetics only partly
mimic the action of endogenous acetylcholine in the hippocampus. They induce theta rhythm as expected but they reduce CA1 pyramidal cell excitability. Our findings are consistent with the assumption that the hippocampal neuronal
cicuitry contains cholinergic synapses that make contact
with interneurons.
In keeping with these findings arecoline moderately impaired LTP. The mechanism and site of action of arecoline to
exert this effect remain to be elucidated.

Topology Related Real-Time Monitoring of Neural Activity in Hippocampal Brain Slices by Noninvasive Optical Recording – A Step Towards Functional Aspects of Long-Term Potentiation (LTP)

P. Saggau and G. ten Bruggencate

Department of Physiology, Universität München, Pettenkoferstrasse 12,
8000 München 2, Federal Republic of Germany

Stimulation induced LTP in guinea pig hippocampal brain slices was monitored in a way to allow direct localization of control and post-tetanic responses with respect to the topology of the neural tissue. To achieve this, optically recorded space- and time-resolved neural activity and videomicrographs of the same area are superimposed on a single display unit during recording. By this method homosynaptic LTP in the CA1-population were demonstrated. Since local LTP-effects can be regarded to be well suited for investigation of fundamental mechanisms of learning and memory within neural populations, this technique facilitates the understanding of the functional properties of this phenomenon.

Being a candidate mechanism for learning and memory, LTP has been intensely investigated in the last decade. One fundamental problem, hindering functional aspects of this phenomenon, was the inability to correlate the topology of the neural population under investigation and its neural activity in real-time. Noninvasive optical recording has proven to be a powerful tool for long-time monitoring neural activity (Saggau et al. 1986) resolved in space and time (Cohen and Lesher 1986; Grinvald 1985; Salzberg 1983). The combination of that technique with modern video-microscopy opens the door to functional aspects of LTP (Saggau and ten Bruggencate 1987).

Transverse slices (300-500 um) of guinea pig hippocampus were held submerged in a perfused optical recording chamber (Saggau et al. 1986). Orthodromic stimulation of strata radiatum (SR) and oriens (SO) was controlled by field potentials recorded in the stratum pyramidale (SP) of the CA1 region. During staining with voltage sensitive fluorescent dyes (e.g. RH 414, 5-20 uM) the perfusion was stopped (20 min) to limit the amount of dye spent per experiment. After re-starting the perfusion and washing out the non bound dye, responses equivalent to the control situation could again be recorded.

Fig. 1A shows the equipment based on an inverted microscope (ZEISS IM 35), employed to measure voltage dependent signals with respect to topology of preparation. Peak-filtered monochromatic light (PF; λ_{ex} = 540 nm) was focussed on to the brain slice (recorded area shaded) via a dichroic mirror (DM) and a x40 objective (OB). Light emitted by fluorescence from a 400 um x 400 um area of the preparation was collected by the objective and, after cut-off filtering (CF; λ_{em} = 610 nm), imaged on two types of photo-detectors by beam-splitting or -switching. For the voltage dependent dye signals a 10 x 10

H. L. Haas   G. Buzsàki (Eds.)
Synaptic Plasticity in the Hippocampus
© Springer-Verlag Berlin Heidelberg 1988

element photodiode-matrix (PDM) in connection with a new type of 100 channel current-to-voltage converter, filter, amplifier and multi-plexer unit (CFA, MUX) was used. The structure of the neural popula-tion under investigation was recorded by a TV-camera (CCD, VID CTRL). All data were collected (A/D), processed (COMP) and displayed (D/A, MON) by a digital computer (DEC LSI-11/23) equipped with an array processor, image processing units and real-world interfaces which controlled the experiment as well.

Fig. 1B demonstrates the facility of the method by showing neural activity elicited by a single orthodromic stimulus given to SR. During the experiment, this spatio-temporal pattern is monitored in real-time, superimposed to an actual videomicrograph of the recorded area.

Fig. 2 illustrates an experiment with noninvasive optical recording of homosynaptic LTP-effects. The spatial resolution was reduced by summing up 2 x 10 PDM-elements to 5 stripes (a-e) 400 um x 80 um each (Fig. 2B), orientated parallel to the CA1-stratification by means of the videomicrograph (Fig. 2C).

Fig. 2A shows the results of a 4-step experiment, the optical recordings being displayed in topology related sequence on top of the electrical field potentials. Responses were elicited by a stimulation of SR (sr) and of SO (so). The first record (AFFERENT VOLLEYS) was performed at the end of the staining period when neural activity, specifically synaptic transmission, was reduced by transient hypoxia. The second record (after resuming perfusion) shows normal activity (CONTROL) and was used as pretetanic reference. The third record (POST

A   B

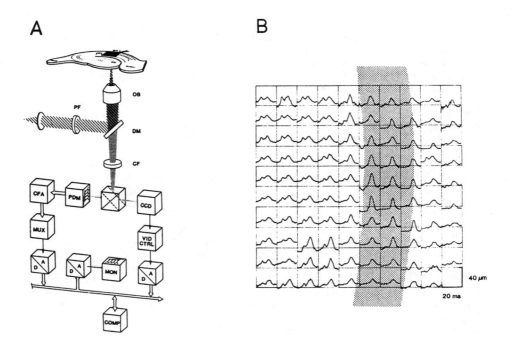

Fig. 1 Principle of recording and visualizing topology-related neural activity. **A** Illustration of the apparatus (abbrev. s. text). **B** Evoked activity (SR left, SP shaded, SO right; 16 sweeps were averaged).

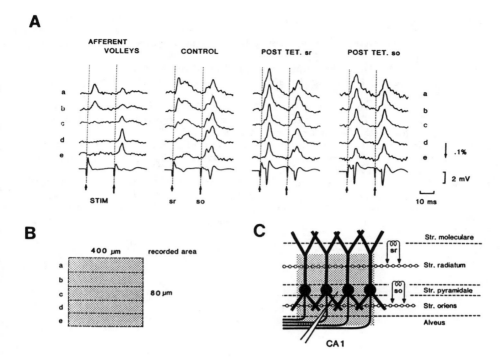

Fig. 2 Optical recording of homosynaptic LTP-effects. **A** Original optical (a-e) and electrical recordings (32 sweeps averaged). Stimulation (abbrev. s. text) is indicated (arrows and dotted lines). **B** Spatial resolution of recorded area. **C** Scheme of CA1-stratification indicating position of electrodes. Optically recorded area shaded.

TET. sr) indicates the responses after brief tetanic stimulation (50 Hz, 2 s, 5 times) of SR. This tetanization lead to a LTP of the sr-response only, leaving the so-response unaltered (note the amplitude of the afferent volleys remaining constant). After tetanizing the SO an equivalent homosynaptic effect was demonstrated for the so-response in the last record (POST TET. so).

The results of the experiments to demonstrate homosynaptic LTP-effects show that noninvasive optical recording of neural activity is well suited to localize such long-lasting changes in synaptic transmission. The ability to correlate local neural activity in real-time with the topology of its substrate allows to attack the analysis of this putative memory related phenomenon.

We thank A. Grinvald and R. Hildesheim for gifts of voltage sensitive dyes. We appreciate the excellent hardware and software support by W. Badke, F. Hahn, R. Hiendl, F. Rucker and G. Wenzel. This work was supported by the DFG (SFB 220) and the Heidenhain-Foundation.

Cohen LB and Lesher S (1986) Optical monitoring of membrane potential; methods of multisite optical measurements. In: De Weer P and Salzberg BM (eds) Optical methods in cell physiology. Wiley, NY USA, pp 71-99

Grinvald A (1985) Real-time optical mapping of neuronal activity: from single growth cones to intact mammalian brain. Ann Rev Neurosci 8: 263-305

Saggau P and ten Bruggencate G (1987) Local long-term potentiation in hippocampal CA1-populations monitored by optical recording of neural activity. Pflügers Arch 408 Suppl 1: R59

Saggau P, Galvan M and ten Bruggencate G (1986) Long-term potentiation in guinea pig hippocampal slices monitored by optical recording of neural activity. Neurosci Lett 69: 53-58

Salzberg BM (1983) Optical recording of electrical activity in neurons using molecular probes. In: Barker JL and McKelvy JF (eds) Current methods in cellular neurobiology. Vol III: Electrophysiological and optical recording techniques. Wiley, NY USA, pp 139-180

Neural Transplants in the Kainic Acid Lesioned Hippocampus: An Investigation of Long-Term Behavioral Effects

U. Sprick and A. Hopf

Institut für Hirnforschung, Universität Düsseldorf, 4000 Düsseldorf,
Federal Republic of Germany

Adult Wistar rats received grafts of embryonic hippocampal tissue
after bilateral neurotoxic lesions of the dorsal hippocampus. The
hippocampal transplants caused an early transient amelioration of
behavioral deficits in a T-maze alternation task and a late long
lasting beneficial effect in the Alkoven Test.

Introduction :

Bilateral kainic acid lesions of the hippocampus   produce
behavioral changes in rats that are mainly characterized by
impairments of maze learning especially in the acquisition of
alternation tasks and locomotor hyperactivity (2). During the
last decade transplants of embryonic neuronal tissue have been
shown to develop fiber connections with the surrounding host
tissue after lesions in various parts of the brain. These
transplants may survive over longer periods of time (1). We
intended to investigate the long-term ability of fetal
hippocampal transplants to reverse behavioral deficits produced
by bilateral hippocampal lesions in adult Wistar rats.

Methods :

Subjects were 35 male adult rats Wistar strain weighing about
250 - 300 grams. They were housed individually under standard
laboratory conditions with free water and food under a 12 / 12
hour dark / light cycle. Three groups of animals were
differentiated :
          group T (N = 15 animals ; lesions plus transplants)
          group L (N = 15 animals ; lesions only)
          group C (N = 5 animals ; controls without lesions)

The animals of group T (N = 15) and group L (N = 15) received
a bilateral lesion of the dorsal hippocampus (coordinates
+2.8 ant.; +2.5 lat.; 2.8 mm dep.;) (5).

0.5 µl kainic acid with a concentration of 1 mg/ml was injected
bilaterally into the dorsal hippocampus under barbiturate
anaesthesia. After the lesions the animals showed the typical
behavioral deficits i.e. general epileptic seizures (ameliorated
by diazepam) as well as stereotyped hyperactive behavior.

One week after the lesion the animals of group T received a
bilateral transplant of embryonic hippocampal tissue, while
animals of group L received a saline injection. For

H. L. Haas   G. Buzsàki (Eds.)
Synaptic Plasticity in the Hippocampus
© Springer-Verlag Berlin Heidelberg 1988

transplantation embryonic hippocampal tissue from day 18 rat
embryos was mechanically homogenated in a 5% glucose solution.
2.0 µl of this solution were injected bilaterally using the same
coordinates which had been used for prior bilateral lesions.

Behavioral testing was started with the Alkoven test. The time
that the animal took to change from the smaller to the larger
compartment was measured in seconds.

The testing was continued in a T-shaped water maze where the
animals had to choose the correct goalarm in an alternation task
(ratio = 3) to escape on a safe platform. There were no
optical clues for the animals to reach the platform because the
platform was just beyond the water surface and could not be
recognized by the swimming rat.

Water maze training began 2 days after transplantation surgery
with shaping sessions for a period of 3 days. The following 12
days the animals had 20 trials daily. The first testing was done
2 weeks after transplantation surgery and continued weekly for 20
weeks. During the test sessions the animals had 20 trials in the
water maze. The number of errors and perseverations were counted.
Perseverations were defined as a block of three false responses
one after the other.

20 weeks after transplantation the animals were perfused and the
brains were histologically examined by various techniques. These
results will be published later.

The test data were statistically processed comparing the mean
values by the Mann-Whitney-U-Test.

Results :

One month after transplantation the animals of group T showed
less mistakes $F(T;1) = 5.4$ and lower perseveration scores
$P(T;1) = 0.4$ than animals of the lesion only group; $F(L;1) = 16.5$
$P(L;1 = 2.6)$. Both differences were significant ($p < 0.05$).
The T-group however still showed impaired test scores in
comparison with the controls. The scores of the controls were
$F(C;1) = 5.1$ and $P(C;1) = 0.2$. The difference between $P(T;1)$ and
$P(C;1)$ was significant ($p < 0.05$).

5 months after transplantation nor the values of mistakes
$F(T;5) = 8.3$ $F(L;5) = 7.9$ neither those of the perseveration
scores $P(T;5) = 1.3$ $P(L;5) = 1.5$ showed significant group
differences between (L) and (T). Fig. 1 shows group
differences of perseveration scores 1 and 5 months after surgery.

These data show an early beneficial transplant effect that did
not persist, however. 5 months after transplantion surgery there
was even a distinct (but nonsignificant) increase in the
number of errors and perseverations in the transplantation group.

In the Alkoven test we found significant group differences
between (L) and (T) 3 months after transplantation,
$A(T;3) = 30.0$ $A(L;3) = 14.3$, while there were no differences
1 month and 5 months after transplantation. The complete Alkoven
values for (L) and (T) were : $A(T;1) = 14.1$, $A(L;1) = 19.7$,
$A(T;5) = 31.7$ and $A(L;5) = 25.3$. Fig. 2 shows group mean values
of the Alkoven test scores.

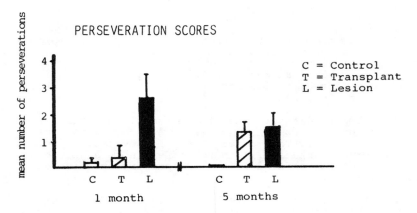

Fig. 1 : group differences of perseveration
          scores 1 and 5 months after surgery

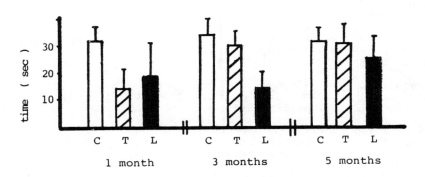

Fig. 2 : group mean values of
          Alkoven Test   scores

These data demonstrate a late persisting benefit effect of the
transplants because the T-group animals achieved significant
higher values 3 months after surgery than the L-group which
reached the same level about 2 months later.   The T-group
persisted on the high score level indicating that this phenomenon
is a long-lasting beneficial effect.

Discussion :

The results confirm the potency of embryonal hippocampal implants for functional recovery after damage of the hippocampus, a structure participating in complex cognition and motoric behaviors (3). Early transient and late long-lasting effects could be differentiated, indicating that the transplants are in mesh with different functional circuits.

These results support data of benefit behavioral effects after transplantation which appeared as late as 9 months after transplantation (4). The increase of perseveration scores 5 months after transplantation, although it was not significant, may be an indicator for some additional maladaptive properties of the transplants.

There are reports in the literature about interfering effects by ingrowth of peripheral catecholaminergic neurones after brain lesions (6).

As we also saw a lot of fibers from surrounding blood vessels sprouting into the transplant and the surrounding host tissue it may be speculated that these fibers interfere with the early amelioration of maze-learning deficits.

Literature :

1.   Bjoerklund A. and Stenevi, U.
      Intracerebral neural implants : neuronal replacement and reconstruction of damaged circuitries.
      ANN. REV. NEUROSCI., 7, 279-308, 1984.

2.   Jarrard, L.E.
      Hippocampal ablation and operant behavior in the rat.
      PSYCHON. SCI. 2, 115-116, 1965.

3.   Kromer, L.F., Bjoerklund, A. and Stenevi, U.
      Regeneration of the septo-hippocampal pathway in adult rats is promoted by utilizing embryonic hippocampal implants as bridges.
      BRAIN RESEARCH, 210, 173-200, 1981.

4.   Pallage, V., Toniolo, G., Will, B. and Hefti, F.
      Long-term effects of nerve growth factor and neural transplants on behavior of rats with medial septal lesions.
      BRAIN RESEARCH, 386, 197-208, 1986.

5.   Pellegrino, L.J., Pellegrino, A.S. and Cushman, A.J.
      A stereotaxic atlas of the rat brain.
      PLENUM PRESS, New York, 1979.

6.   Stenevi, U. and Björklund, A.
      Growth of vascular sympathetic axons into the hippocampus after lesions of the septo-hippocampal pathway: a pitfall in brain lesion studies.
      NEUROSCI. LET., 7, 219-224, 1978.

Kindling and Epilepsy

Calcium Binding Proteins and Experimental Models of Epilepsy

K. G. BAIMBRIDGE and J. J. MILLER

Department of Physiology, University of British Columbia, Vancouver, BC V6t 1W5, Canada

The function of two calcium binding proteins, Calbindin D28k and Parvalbumin has been examined in the kindled rat and genetically epileptic (El) mouse. Calbindin D28k is reduced in specific areas of both animal models of epilepsy while Parvalbumin is greatly elevated, (particularly in cortical regions), of the El mouse.

Calcium has been implicated in the mechanisms of both long-term potentiation and kindling. The high frequency stimuli required for both these processes result in a large influx of calcium into the postsynatic site (1). On entering the neuron calcium may interact with an increasingly wide variety of intracellular proteins which have an affinty for calcium in the micromolar range. Calmodulin and calcineurin have specific enzyme activator functions while others such as calbindin D28k (CaBP) and parvalbumin (PV) have been suggested to be intraneuronal calcium buffering systems(2). Within the hippocampus CaBP is present in the dentate granule (DG) and a sub-population of CA1 pyramidal cells. The CA3 pyramidal cells have no CaBP(3). PV is found throughout the hippocampal formation in a sub-population of GABAergic neurons closely associated with the principal neurons and is found in almost all cortical GABAergic neurons (6).

We have been studying changes in CaBP and PV associated with two animal models of epilepsy, kindling and the El mouse. In the rat kindling stimuli delivered to any of a number of different sites results in a progressive decline in the levels of CaBP specifically within the DG cells. The lowest CaBP levels are reached just prior to the onset of full motor seizures and are maintained for weeks without further kindling stimuli (4,5,11). Six months after establishing seizures, however, CaBP levels have returned to normal even though re-stimulation results in seizures on the first or second trial.

Aside from the changes in CaBP a number of other biochemical correlates of kindling have been identified specifically within the DG cells. These include changes in the phosphorylation state of membrane proteins (19) the benzodiazepine receptor (15) and a loss of dynorphin immunoreactivity (Dyn-IR) (13). We consider that these extensive changes are not necessarily causal to the maintenance of kindling but that they may either be important in establishing seizures or be a events designed to counteract epileptiform activity in the hiippocampus. In the latter respect the important feature may be the central function of the dentate gyrus in regulating the flow of information

H.L. Haas   G. Buzsàki (Eds.)
Synaptic Plasticity in the Hippocampus
© Springer-Verlag Berlin Heidelberg 1988

from the cortex to the CA3 pyramidal cells; an area known to be prone to aberrant discharge.

The functional consequences of the loss of CaBP could be many and varied. Essentially one might predict that the loss of a major intracellualr buffering system could have profound effects on any process regulated by an increase in intracellur calcium. These include biochemical mechanisms induced by a calcium-calmodulin type interaction, the calcium dependent late potassium conductance, the entry of calcium from the extracellular environment or neurotransmitter release. To the extent that it has been studied the electrophysiological studies have shown that "kindled" DG cells have an enhanced paired pulse inhibition (16,18), much more pronounced dendritic calcium spikes and greatly enhanced stimulus induced calcium fluxes (see Mody, this volume). No attention has yet been paid to the possible influence of CaBP in regulating the output of DG cells possibly via an interaction with neurotransmitter release.

The reduction of Dyn-IR seen in the kindled rat appears to require seizure activity and is short lived in that normal levels are re-established within four weeks in the absence of further kindling stimuli. The function of dynorphin in the mossy fiber terminals is unknown but it is interesting to note that, although stimulation of the mossy fibers produces an excitatory effect on CA3 pyramidal cells, the effect of dynorphin appears to be predominantly one of inhibition (9). In the peripheral nervous system evidence has been accumulated by Lundberg and his colleagues (11) for the frequency dependent differential release of a classical transmitter co-existing with a peptide neurotransmitter/neuromodulator. It is possible therefore that dynorphin is only released under conditions of high frequency stimulation and that in these circumstances it may act to prevent excessive activity in the CA3 region.

A model will be presented which proposes that one of the functions of CaBP may be to regulate the frequency dependent differential release of co-existing transmitters by a tight regulation of intraterminal free calcium concentration. The loss of CaBP would result in a loss of this regulatory process and the release of dynorphin at lower frequency of stimulation. The combined effect would therefore be an alteration in neurotransmitter release from the mossy fiber bouton which would be both quantitative and qualitative in nature and serve to resist the development of seizures.

The E1 mouse was originally developed in Japan and is characterized by the induction of seizures through mild vestibular stimulation. The neurochemical findings to date indicate a reduced level of whole brain norepinephrine, and significant elevations in brain ACh, taurine and GABA (9,10). Additionally our own studies have shown decreased CaBP levels in the hippocampal formation and distinct cortical regions (14). The presence of PV within GABAergic neurons (6) has given us the opportunity to assess theses neurons indirectly by assaying regional brain PV levels in E1 and control (Swiss) mice.

The induction of seizures in the E1 mice has been described in detail elsewhere (14) and the same tissue processing was used to generate soluble protein fractions. Control and El mice (weight range 28–40 gm) were sacrificed and their entire brain removed as rapidly as possible and dissected into the following regions: dorsal parietal, ventral temporal, dorsal and ventral occipital cortex (DPC, DTC, DOC and VOC); hippocampal formation (HF), striatum (Str), medulla (Med), cerebellum, pons and midbrain. The tissue was homogenised and the soluble protein fraction used for PV determination by radioimmunoassay. Animals of both sexes were used in this study and since no sex differences were noted (unlike that of CaBP) the data has been pooled. The results are shown in Fig 1.

With the exception of the VOC all cortical regions of the El mice had greatly elevated levels of PV (up to 170% above controls). In addition PV was also elevated in the medulla and striatum but was not significantly different from control values in the HF, cerebellum, pons or midbrain. It is interesting to note that the elevated cortical levels of PV were found in precisely the same regions in which CaBP levels were previously shown to be decreased (14). Immunohistochemical studies are now underway to determine whether or not the increase in PV is an increased concentration within the PV–GABA neurons or an actual increased number of neurons. The latter effect has been observed in another animal model of epilepsy, the seizure sensitive gerbil, in which an increase in the number of GAD-postive neurons was found specifically associated with the dentate granule cell layer of the hippocampal formation (17).

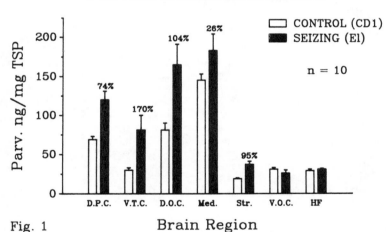

Fig. 1   Brain Region

References

1. Baimbridge K.G. and Miller J.J. Brain Res. 221: 299-305,1981
2. Baimbridge K.G. et al Brain Res. 239:519-525,1982
3. Baimbridge K.G. and Miller J.J. Brain Res. 245: 223-229,1982
4. Baimbridge K.G. and Miller J.J. Brain Res. 324:85-90,1984
5. Baimbridge K.G., Mody I and Miller J.J. Epilepsia 26:460-465,1985
6. Celio M.R. Science 231:995-997,1986
7. Heizmann C.W. Experientia 40:910-921,1984
8. Henriksen S.J, Chouvet G. and Bloom F.E. Life Sci. 31:1785-88,1982
9. Iwata H. et al Jap. J.Pharmacol 29:503-507,1979
10. Kurokawa M. et al Prog Brain Res. 21A:112-130,1966
11. Lundberg J.M. and Hokfelt T. TINS 6:325-333,1983
12. Miller J.J. and Baimbridge K.G. Brain Res 278:322-326,1983
13. McGinty J.F et al Neuroscience Letters 71: 31-36,1986
14. Mody I., Baimbridge K.G. and Miller J.J. Epilep. Res.1:46-52,1987
15. Niznik H.B. Burnham W.M. and Kish S.J. J.Neurochem 43:1732-36,1984
16. Oliver M.W. and Miller J.J. Exp. Brain Res. 57: 443-447,1985
17. Peterson G.M. et al Brain Res. 340:384-389,1985
18. Tuff L.P., Racine R.J. and Adamec R. Brain Res. 277:79-90,1983
19. Wasterlain C.G. and Farber D.B. Brain Res. 247:191-194,1982

Long-Term Modifications of Hippocampal Function Following Chronic Experimental Epilepsy

J. G. R. JEFFERYS

Department of Physiology and Biophysics, St. Mary's Hospital Medical School,
London W2 1PG, United Kingdom

Injecting a small dose of tetanus toxin into rat hippocampus
establishes an epileptic focus which generates seizures which recur
intermittently for the subsequent 4-8 weeks. The seizures eventually
cease but the rats retain permanent impairments in learning and
memory, even though no histopathology has been found in this model.
Therefore we explored the physiological changes that might be
involved. The principal results were that LTP appeared to be intact,
but that postsynaptic responses from the pyramidal cell of CA1 and
CA3a were depressed for at least 8 months afterwards.

The intrahippocampal tetanus toxin syndrome in rat provides a chronic
experimental epilepsy with a special relevance to limbic epilepsies
(temporal lobe epilepsy/partial complex seizures); both to the
mechanism of the seizures themselves, and to the behavioural problems
that can occur at other times (Mellanby et al 1977, 1984). The
primary effect of the toxin probably is to block synaptic inhibition
by disrupting the release of GABA (Collingridge et al, 1981).

In our experiments we made stereotaxic injections of 5 mouse LD_{50} of
tetanus toxin, in 0.5 ul of buffer, into the hippocampi of rats
anaesthetized with Sagatal. The rats were kept for varying intervals
after recovery before terminal experiments were performed to study
hippocampal electrophysiology. In general, the active focus was
examined using the slice preparation in vitro, <30 days after
injection; the long-term changes have so far been studied under
halothane anaesthesia in vivo >8 weeks after injection.

The active focus

Epileptic discharges were preserved in 400 μm thick hippocampal slices
prepared from rats 3-30 days after injection (Jefferys, 1986). The
focus appeared to mature over the first 2 weeks or so. Initially
slices generated epileptiform afterdischarges in response to
electrical stimulation. With longer survival times (>7 days) they
also generated spontaneous epileptic bursts which were associated with
"paroxysmal depolarization shifts" in intracellular recordings. These
bursts occurred rather infrequently, typically once every few minutes,
but when they occurred they could last several seconds. The extent of
neuronal synchronization during these epileptic bursts was very
variable, both in terms of the amplitude of the bursts and the
distance of propagation. The variability of bursts in any single

H. L. Haas   G. Buzsàki (Eds.)
Synaptic Plasticity in the Hippocampus
© Springer-Verlag Berlin Heidelberg 1988

slice may well be due to residual functional inhibitory synapses. With survival times in excess of 3 weeks it appeared that the propagation of bursts was progressively restricted to the centre of the focus, implicating other processes, which perhaps provide an adaptive response to the chronic seizures, and which may represent the onset of the neuronal depression which is one of the principal long-term effects of the toxin. Slices prepared 8 weeks after injection generated no epileptiform activity, and while quantitative studies are required, I formed the impression that these slices were less excitable than normal.

Long-term effects of tetanus toxin

8-10 weeks after injection, all seizures have ceased. This period is particularly interesting as, in the absence of any known histopathology (Mellanby et al, 1977; Kessler and Markowitz, 1983), there are permanent impairments on a range of behavioural tasks, particularly involving learning and memory. In order to explore the physiological mechanisms responsible for these long-term consequences we used terminal experiments under halothane anaesthesia.

Our initial hypothesis had been that there was a specific impairment of long-term potentiation. However, LTP in CA3a proved to be intact, at least over periods of up to 5 hours. These experiments did reveal significant and consistent changes. Postsynaptic population spikes recorded from CA3a and CA1 were depressed, which, with the presentation of the evoked potentials corresponding to the synaptic currents and to antidromic spikes, suggest that these pyramidal cells had a decreased excitability. Curiously, CA3c appeared to be resistant to these long-term changes, even though this subregion had clearly been affected by the toxin, being the site of initiation of the epileptic bursts in at least some slices obtained 7 to 30 days after injection (Brace et al, 1985; Jefferys and Williams, 1985, 1987, submitted). Mellanby and Sundstrum (1986) have reported that the dentate granule cells were similarly affected.

The mechanisms responsible for these long-term changes in neuronal responses remain to be resolved. Inhibition was either normal (feed-forward) or remained weakened (recurrent), so that a re-active increase in the number or efficiency of inhibitory synapses remains unlikely (Williams and Jefferys, 1985; Jefferys and Williams, submitted). Neurochemical markers for a range of neurotransmitters were also normal (Bowen, Francis and Jefferys, in preparation). At present we would speculate that the changes are in the intrinsic excitability of the principal neurones themselves. There is some circumstantial evidence implicating mechanisms involving protein kinase C or inositol triphosphate, because these appear to be concentrated in the hippocampal regions which exhibited the greatest long-term effects of tetanus toxin.

This work was supported by the Wellcome Trust, the Medical Research Council and the Thorn Trust. The author is a Wellcome Trust Senior Lecturer.

REFERENCES

Brace HM, Jefferys JGRJ & Mellanby J. Long-term changes in
hippocampal physiology and learning ability of rats after
intrahippocampal tetanus toxin. Journal of Physiology 1985; 368:
343-357.

Collingridge GL, Thompson PA, Davies J & Mellanby J. In vitro effect
of tetanus toxin on release of GABA from hippocampal slices. Journal
of Neurochemistry 1981; 37: 1039-1041.

Jefferys JGR. Tetanus toxin chronic epileptic foci in rat hippocampal
slices. Journal of Physiology 1986; 373: 24P.

Jefferys JGR & Williams SF. Physiological and behavioural
consequences of seizures induced in the rat by intrahippocampal
tetanus toxin. Brain 1987; 110: 517-532.

Jefferys JGR & Williams SF. Long-term depression of CA3 hippocampal
neurones following intrahippocampal injection of tetanus toxin in
rats. Journal of Physiology 1985; 360: 33P.

Kessler J & Markowitsch HJ. Different neuropathological effects of
intrahippocampal injections of kainic acid and tetanus toxin.
Experientia 1983; 39: 922-924.

Mellanby J, George G, Robinson A & Thompson P. Epileptiform syndrome
in rats produced by injecting tetanus toxin into the hippocampus.
Journal of Neurology, Neurosurgery and Psychiatry 1977; 40: 404-414.

Mellanby J, Hawkins C, Mellanby H, Rawlins JNP & Impey ME. Tetanus
toxin as a tool for studying epilepsy. Journal de Physiologie 1984;
Paris 79: 207-215.

Mellanby JH & Sundstrom L. Long-term reduction in excitability of rat
dentate granule cells after tetanus toxin. Journal of Physiology
1986; 371: 49P.

Williams SF & Jefferys JGR. Inhibition and long-term neuronal
depression after intra-hippocampal tetanus toxin. Neuroscience
Letters 1985; supplement 22: S510.

Activation of NMDA Receptors in the Dentate Gyrus Following Kindling-Induced Epilepsy

I. MODY

Playfair Neuroscience Unit, Toronto Western Hospital, 399 Bathurst St. Toronto, Ontario M5T 2S8, Canada

The N-methyl-D-aspartate (NMDA) receptors, although present in high density on granule cells (GCs) of the rat dentate gyrus[1] (DG), do not normally contribute to low frequency synaptic transmission through the perforant pathway[2]. Following kindling-induced epilepsy however, these receptors become involved in the generation of postsynaptic potentials[3]. In granule cells, the altered synaptic properties induced by kindling are long-lasting and are paralleled by significant changes in the electrical properties of the neuronal membrane, that may both lead to the generation of epileptiform activity.

In the dentate gyrus, repetitive stimulation of afferent fibers produces plastic, long-lasting neuronal alterations. Short duration, high frequency stimuli induce long-term potentiation[4] (LTP) of synaptic transmission, but if the stimulation is repeated daily, generalized convulsions will result (kindling[5]). This paradigm is widely used as a model of experimental epilepsy[6]. Although several neurochemical and electrophysiological correlates of kindling-induced epilepsy have been described in the central nervous system[7], the basic underlying mechanisms remain obscure. The present study is based on the recognition of the DG as the site of many kindling-related alterations[8] and the involvement of NMDA receptors in several other models of neuronal plasticity and experimental epilepsy[9]. The findings demonstrate that in contrast to controls, GCs in hippocampal slices prepared from kindled animals display an NMDA receptor-mediated component in synaptic transmission[11]. Furthermore, kindling produces significant alterations in the membrane characteristics of GCs.

The cellular and synaptic properties of GCs were examined using intra-/extracellular and Ca^{2+}-sensitive microelectrode recordings following kindling through the hippocampal commissures or amygdala. The recordings were made in hippocampal slices prepared from sham-stimulated controls and animals that reached stage IV-V[10] of kindling. The mean number of stimulation trials (60 Hz/1 s, 100-150 μA) required to reach full motor seizures (stage V) were 23 ± 2 for commissural kindling and 14 ± 1 for amygdala kindling. The resting membrane potential of GCs following kindling (RMP; -72 ± 3 mV), was not significantly different from the RMP of control GCs (-70 ± 2 mV). Similarly, action potential height and threshold were unaffected by kindling. However, other cellular properties of GCs changed regardless of the site of stimulation, the stage of kindling reached (IV or V), or the time elapsed between the last kindling stimulus and preparation of hippocampal slices (24 hrs to 6 weeks). The input resistance (R_N) of kindled GCs (55 ± 4 MΩ) was significantly higher than that of

H.L. Haas   G. Buzsàki (Eds.)
Synaptic Plasticity in the Hippocampus
© Springer-Verlag Berlin Heidelberg 1988

control GCs (40 ± 3 MΩ). In contrast to most control GCs, the slope conductance (G_s) of kindled neurons, measured with constant amplitude current pulses injected at various membrane potentials, generally increased at membrane potentials more negative than rest. Furthermore, ionic conductances (Ca^{2+}-spikes and possibly a persistent Na^+ current; see below), that were not normally encountered in control GCs, were present in kindled neurons.

The intracellularly recorded monosynaptic excitatory postsynaptic potentials (EPSPs) of kindled GCs, evoked through the stimulation of the lateral perforant pathway, differed significantly from the EPSPs of control GCs (Fig.1).

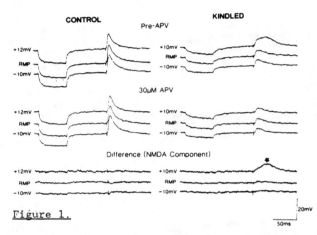

Figure 1.

The amplitudes of control EPSPs increased upon membrane hyperpolarizations and decreased following depolarizations, as expected for conventional EPSPs without contribution from voltage-dependent conductances. In contrast, the EPSPs of kindled GCs invariably increased in amplitude and duration at membrane potentials 5-20 mV depolarized from RMP, indicating the presence of a voltage-dependent component. Perfusion of the NMDA receptor antagonist DL-2-amino-5-phosphonovaleric acid (APV; 30 μM) had no effect on the EPSPs of control GCs, but consistently reduced the amplitude and duration of EPSPs in kindled GCs. In kindled neurons, but not in controls, digital subtraction of EPSPs recorded in the presence of APV from EPSPs evoked before APV perfusion revealed a clear APV-sensitive component in synaptic transmission. This component appears to be mediated by NMDA receptors, and is most likely due to the increased conductance of the associated channels at these potentials. Omission of extracellular Mg^{2+} ($[Mg^{2+}]_o$) from the perfusate, in order to remove the voltage-dependent block from NMDA gated channels[9], had different effects on control and kindled GCs. In control cells, perfusion of Mg^{2+}-free medium reduced action potential threshold by 2-8 mV without affecting EPSPs or RMP. In contrast, the absence of $[Mg^{2+}]_o$ hyperpolarized kindled GCs by 5-8 mV and produced large increases in EPSP amplitudes triggering bursts of action potentials. These effects were reversibly antagonized by APV, showing that NMDA receptor activation was, at least in part, responsible for the altered synaptic properties of kindled GCs in low $[Mg^{2+}]_o$.

In both kindled and control GCs, intracellular injections of the lidocaine derivative QX 314 (50 mM) blocked fast Na^+ spikes and depolarized the membrane by 15-20 mV probably due to the inhibition of a steady state K^+ conductance (Fig.2A&B). Following cessation of fast Na^+ action potentials, slow spikes, presumably mediated by Ca^{2+}, could be evoked in kindled GCs with depolarizing current pulses (Fig.2B), steady depolarizations of the membrane, or synaptic stimulation when

178

the cells were held at depolarized membrane potentials. In contrast, blockade of Na$^+$ action potentials by QX 314 in control GCs was never sufficient to evoke slow Ca^{2+} spikes (Fig.2A). Perfusion of APV (30 μM) selectively blocked the synaptically evoked Ca^{2+} spikes of kindled GCs, but had no effect on Ca^{2+} spikes evoked by depolarizing current pulses. Thus, the depolarizations produced by synaptic activation of NMDA receptors were effective in triggering Ca^{2+} spikes.

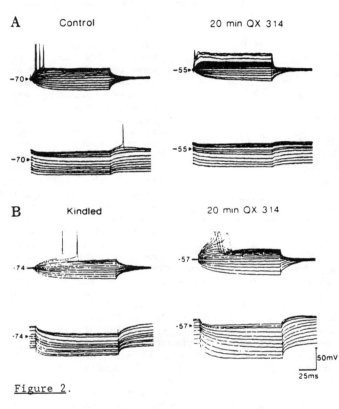

A   Control   20 min QX 314

B   Kindled   20 min QX 314

Figure 2.

Intracellular QX 314 also reduced the G_s of kindled GCs, but not that of controls, possibly due to the presence of a persistent inward Na$^+$ conductance specific only to kindled neurons.

Recordings with Ca^{2+}-sensitive microelectrodes revealed that decreases in extracellular Ca^{2+} ($\Delta[Ca^{2+}]_o$) evoked by repetitive stimulation (20 Hz/10 s) of the perforant pathway were significantly larger in kindled dentate gyri than in controls. Frequently, in the kindled dentate, repetitive stimulation evoked spreading depression (SD) associated with large (>1.2 mM) $\Delta[Ca^{2+}]_o$ and 10-15 mV shifts in field potentials. Such SDs could not be evoked in the dentate gyri of control slices bathed in normal perfusate, even with high intensity repetitive stimulation[11].

The present data show long-lasting alterations in cellular and synaptic properties of kindled GCs, and reveal that the recruitment of NMDA receptors in synaptic transmission may be an important functional correlate of plastic neuronal changes.

Supported by MRC of Canada and Killam Fellowships to I.M. and DFG Grants to U. Heinemann.

REFERENCES :

1. Monaghan, D.T. & Cotman, C.W., J. Neurosci., 5: 2909-2919, 1985.

2. Crunelli, V. & al., J. Physiol., 341: 627-640, 1983.

3. Mody, I. & Heinemann, U., Nature, 326: 701-704, 1987.

4. Bliss, T.V.P. & Gardner-Medwin, A.R., J. Physiol., 232: 357-374, 1973; Bliss, T.V.P. & Lomo, T., J. Physiol., 232: 334-356, 1973.

5. Goddard, G.V., Nature, 214: 1020-1021, 1967.

6. Racine, R., Neurosurgery, 3: 234-252, 1978; McNamara, J.O. & al., Progr. Neurobiol., 15: 139-159, 1980.

7. Kalichman, M.W., Neurosci. Biobehav. Rev., 6: 161-181, 1982

8. Tuff, L.P. & al., Brain Res., 277: 79-90, 1983; Oliver, M.W. & Miller, J.J., Exp. Brain Res., 57: 443-447, 1985; Baimbridge, K.G., this issue.

9. Mayer, M.L. & Westbrook, G.L., Progr. Neurobiol., 28: 197-276, 1987.

10. Racine, R., Electroenceph. clin. Neurophysiol., 32: 281-294, 1972.

11. Mody, I. & al., J. Neurophysiol., 57: 869-888, 1987.

Regenerative, All-or-None, Electrographic Seizures in the Rat Hippocampal Slice in Physiological Magnesium Medium*

W. W. Anderson, H. S. Swartzwelder, and W. A. Wilson

Departments of Pharmacology, Medicine and Psychology, Duke University, and Epilepsy Center, V.A. Medical Center, Durham, NC 27706, USA

Previous studies have shown that electrographic seizures (EGSs) can occur spontaneously for several hours in the hippocampal slice in Mg-free medium containing the GABA$_b$ agonist baclofen. We report here that similar all-or-none EGSs could be triggered in physiological Mg medium (with or without baclofen) if the EGSs were induced by several stimulus trains, and sometimes transiently exposed to Mg-free medium.

EGSs can be induced in brain slices by a wide variety of chemical manipulations. Removal of Mg from the extracellular medium induces spontaneous EGSs of about 50 sec duration in CA3 of the rat hippocampal slice, and, if baclofen is added, can persist for several hours [1,7]. Mg-free medium also induces EGSs in slices from the entorhinal cortex [8] and neocortex [2]. EGSs have also been produced in brain slices by low Cl, low Ca, high K, penicillin, bicuculline, and 4-aminopyridine (see Refs in [7]). In physiological medium, EGSs have been recorded in pyriform cortex slices from kindled animals [4]. However, to our knowledge, there are no reports of seizure-like events in brain slices from naive animals in physiological medium. Here we report hippocampal slices from naive animals given repeated stimulus trains in physiological medium containing baclofen, or additional brief exposure to Mg-free medium, subsequently express all-or-none EGSs in physiological medium (with or without baclofen).

Slices (625 uM thick) were prepared from male Sprague-Dawley rats (25-37 days old). Normal medium contained (in mM): NaCl 120, KCl 3.3, NaHCO$_3$ 25, NaH$_2$PO$_4$ 1.23, dextrose 11, and either 0.9/1.3 or 1.2/1.8 MgSO$_4$/CaCl$_2$. Rat CSF contains 0.88 mM Mg [3]. Mg-free medium was prepared by omitting MgSO$_4$. Extracellular recording and stimulation were conducted in s. pyramidale and s. radiatum of CA3, respectively. The stimulus amplitude (15-50 V or 150-400 uA, .1 msec) was twice that used to obtain the maximum orthodromic population spike amplitude. The threshold for seizure initiation was tested by delivering stimulus trains of either constant (2 sec) duration and variable pulse frequency, or constant (60 Hz) pulse frequency and variable duration.

---

* Supported by the Veterans Administration and NIH Grant NS-17771.

H. L. Haas G. Buzsàki (Eds.)
Synaptic Plasticity in the Hippocampus
© Springer-Verlag Berlin Heidelberg 1988

In Mg-free medium containing 2-5 uM baclofen, most slices produced spontaneous EGSs. In slices which did not, a single stimulus pulse or a weak train (2 sec, 3-10 pulses) triggered an EGS. In either case, a much stronger stimulus train (2 sec, 120 pulses) triggered a nearly identical EGS. The EGSs in Mg-free medium + baclofen were all-or-none events with a distinct triggering threshold.

We then attempted to obtain stimulus train triggered, all-or-none EGSs in physiological medium by using repeated stimulus trains to induce stimulus train generated afterdischarges (ADs) [6], and then testing for all-or none behavior. When slices were placed in medium containing 0.9-1.2 mM Mg, and 0.5-5 uM baclofen (to supress interictal-like bursts), delivery of stimulus trains (2 sec, 60 Hz, once every 10 min) induced progressively longer ADs. Usually only a few AD bursts occurred following the first stimulus train, and the maximum ADs were reached at 3-10 trains. This indicates that AD induction occurred as a result of the trains.

After the ADs were induced, stimulus trains of variable duration or pulse frequency were delivered in the same medium to test the all-or-none nature of the ADs (Fig. 1). The all-or-none response is defined as no AD bursts at subthreshold stimulations, and a constant AD duration at all suprathreshold stimulations. Some slices did not produce unambiguous all-or-none ADs after more than 10 stimulus trains in 0.9-1.2 uM Mg + baclofen, but did so following an additional 0.5 hr exposure to Mg-free medium. Five of 10 slices from 10 animals produced unambiguous all-or-none ADs in 0.9-1.2 mM Mg following induction by this protocol. ADs were 20-30 sec long and required 17-56 pulses for triggering. One of these slices also produced all-or-none ADs in medium containing 1.2 mM Mg and no baclofen, indicating that baclofen does not have to be present to obtain all-or-none ADs. Furthermore, 2 slices exhibited near all-or-none behavior, producing only 1 and 2 AD bursts at subthreshold stimulations. The other 3 slices showed a continuum of AD burst number and duration.

These results demonstrate that all-or-none ADs can be obtained in normal Mg (with or without baclofen) following induction by stimulus trains or additional exposure to Mg-free medium. Because these all-or-none ADs are very similar to the spontaneous and triggered EGSs occurring in Mg-free medium (except for a higher threshold and shorter duration), they can be considered EGSs. Factors which may be important for obtaining these all-or-none EGSs include using young animals, having a minimum of interictal-like bursting (by using baclofen), and using long intervals between stimulus trains (unpublished observations). Because these EGSs are induced by stimulus trains and have a distinct trigger threshold, they are phenomenologically similar to EGSs induced and triggered by stimulus trains in animals during kindling [5]. The all-or-none EGS response indicates that the EGS cannot simply be generated by a long duration EPSP, but implies the involvement of one or more regenerative mechanisms.

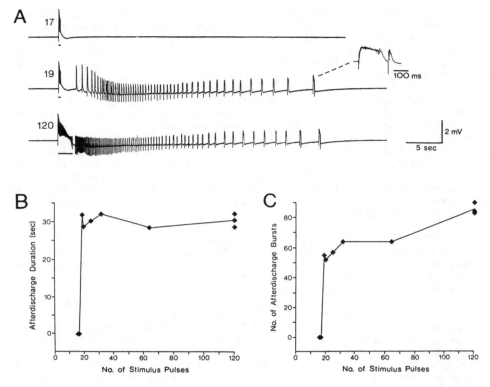

Fig. 1. All-or-none EGSs in 0.9 mM Mg medium + 2 uM baclofen triggered by 60 Hz stimulus trains of different durations. The slice received 10 trains (2 sec, 60 Hz) prior to the test trains. A) 19 and 120 pulses triggered ADs of nearly identical durations; 17 pulses did not trigger any AD bursts. B) Graphs of the AD duration (in sec) and C) the number of AD bursts, versus the number of pulses in a train.

References

1 Anderson WW, Lewis DV, Swartzwelder HS, Wilson WA (1986) Magnesium-free medium activates seuzure-like events in the rat hippocampal slice. Brain Res 398: 215-219

2 Aram JA, Lodge D (1987) Effects of anticonvulsants on NMDA receptor-mediated epileptiform activity in rat cortical slices superfused with Mg^{2+}-free medium. Brit J Pharm 90: 6P

3 Chutkow JG, Meyers S (1968) Chemical changes in the cerebrospinal fluid and brain in magnesium deficiency. Neurology 18: 963-974

4 McIntyre DC, Wong RKS (1985) Modification of local neuronal interactions by amygdala kindling examined in vitro. Exp Neurol 88: 529-537

5 McNamara JO, Bonhaus DW, Shin C, Crain BJ, Gellman RL, Giacchino JL
   (1985) The kindling model of epilepsy: a critical review. CRC Crit
   Rev Clin Neurobiol 1: 341-391.

6 Stasheff SF, Bragdon AC, Wilson WA (1985) Induction of
   epileptiform activity in hippocampal slices by trains of
   electrical stimuli. Brain Res 344: 296-302

7 Swartzwelder HS, Lewis DV, Anderson WW, Wilson WA (1987) Seizure-
   like events in brain slices: Supression by spontaneous interictal
   spikes. Brain Res in press

8 Walther H, Lambert JDC, Jones RSG, Heinemann U, Hamon B (1986)
   Epileptiform activity in combined slices of the hippocampus,
   subiculum and entorhinal cortex during perfusion with low magnesium
   medium. Neurosci Lett 69: 156-161

Altered Noradrenergic Modulation of Dentate Granule Cell Firing and N-Methyl-D-Aspartate (NMDA) Receptors After Kindlung

P.K. STANTON, I. MODY[1], and U. HEINEMANN[2]

Department of Biophysics, Johns Hopkins University, Baltimore, MD 21218, USA; [1]Playfair Neuroscience Unit, Toronto, Ontario M5T 2S8, Canada; and [2]Institute for Normal and Pathologic Physiology, Universität Köln, 5000 Köln, Federal Republic of Germany

Abstract: Depleting brain norepinephrine (NE) impairs long-term potentiation (LTP) of perforant path (PP)-dentate gyrus (DG) synapses, promotes induction of kindled epilepsy, and NE elicits long-lasting potentiation of PP evoked potentials. We now report that NE enhances both stimulus and NMDA induced Ca^{2+} influx into granule cells via β_1 receptors, and elicits long-lasting depolarization requiring NMDA receptor activation to persist. Furthermore, the induction of kindled epilepsy is associated with reduced sensitivity to NE, which may represent a neuronal "write-protect" mechanism and also contribute to epileptogenesis.

There is mounting evidence of an important role for the monoamine neurotransmitter norepinephrine (NE) in the expression of long-term central nervous system plasticity. Locus coeruleus stimulation can modulate learned task performance[1] and increase the synaptic efficacy of the perforant path (PP) input to the dentate gyrus (DG),[2]. Depletion of forebrain NE has been shown to interfere with induction of long-term potentiation (LTP) at PP-DG synapses[3], and accelerate the induction of kindled epilepsy[4], and exogenous NE induces LTP of PP evoked potentials[5].

At the same time, growing evidence indicates that glutamate receptors of the N-methyl-D-aspartate (NMDA) subtype are also important to expression of LTP and kindled epilepsy. NMDA receptor antagonists block production of LTP[6] and retard kindling[7] when present during high-frequency stimulation.

In light of these findings, we employed ion-selective, extra- and intracellular recordings in the in vitro hippocampal slice, to study noradrenergic modulation of dentate gyrus plasticity, with respect to (1) actions of NE on granule cell response to high-frequency stimulation, (2) activity-independent long-lasting effects of NE on granule cells, (3) interactions between NE and NMDA-mediated responses and (4) effects of prior induction of kindling on the actions of NE on granule cells.

Hippocampal slices (400-450 μm thick) were prepared by standard methods[8] and maintained in a modified Haas interface perfusion chamber[9]. Extracellular/ion-selective double barreled electrodes were prepared as described elsewhere[10], and 4 M K Acetate electrodes (R=50-120 MΩ) were used for intracellular recordings. For kindling, male Wistar rats (180-220 g; n=30) were stereotactically implanted under Na-pentobarbital anaesthesia, either in the hippocampal commissures[11] or the amygdaloid nucleus[12]. After 7-10 days recovery, kindled rats were stimulated daily (60 Hz/1 s; 100-150 μA) until 5 consecutive stage V seizures[13] were elicited. Twenty-four hours to 6 weeks after the last stimuli, slices were prepared as usual and compared to slices from sham-operated controls (n=10).

Bath applying NE (50 μM) markedly enhanced both Ca^{2+} influx and K^+ efflux evoked by high-frequency PP stimulation of a type which elicits LTP (20 Hz/10 s). This effect was reversible, and blocked by the β_1 antagonist metoprolol. Furthermore, we found that the NMDA receptor antagonist 2-amino-5-phosphonovalerate (APV 30 μM) also blocked noradrenergic enhancement of stimulus-evoked Ca^{2+} influx. This led us to test the actions of NE on Ca^{2+} influx induced by iontophoresing

H.L. Haas   G. Buzsàki (Eds.)
Synaptic Plasticity in the Hippocampus
© Springer-Verlag Berlin Heidelberg 1988

excitatory amino acids onto granule cells. In these experiments, NE produced a marked potentiation of NMDA-induced Ca^{2+} influx, while not affecting Ca^{2+} influx induced by quisqualic acid.

We next attempted, through intracellular recordings, to find what persistent effects of NE on granule neurons might correlate with long-term plasticity. NE depolarized granule cells with an increase in input resistance (R_N), blocked accomodation of firing to depolarizing current injection or synaptic tetanus, and blocked the late burst- induced afterhyperpolarization (AHP) - all actions antagonized by metoprolol. NE also produced an α_1 receptor mediated block of regenerative Ca^{2+} potentials (after injecting Cs^+ to block K^+ currents and QX314 to block Na^+ spikes). Interestingly, the depolarization and increase in R_N were both long-lasting after washout of NE, similar to long-lasting potentiation of PP evoked population potentials elicited by NE.

In further studies addressing the role of NMDA receptors in NE-induced plasticity, we found that the NMDA receptor antagonist APV (30 µM) specifically blocked both the NE-induced potentiation of PP evoked population potentials, as well as blocking the long-lasting phase of depolarization and R_N increase recorded intracellularly. Taken together, these findings support the conclusion that NE modulates granule cell long-term plasticity via β_1 receptor activation, leading to activation of normally quiescent NMDA receptors.

We have also looked for alterations in noradrenergic actions following induction of kindled epilepsy. Kindling is an example of long-term plasticity induced by daily high-frequency stimulation leading, within days or weeks, to the establishment of a chronic epileptic focus that may be active for many months[14]. Like LTP, kindling is blocked by NMDA receptor antagonists[7]. Kindling has also been shown to be associated with enhanced participation of NMDA receptors in dentate synaptic transmission[15]. Therefore, we compared actions of NE on granule cells in slices taken from kindled rats with the known noradrenergic effects we observed in control untetanized slices.

After the induction of kindled epilepsy, we found significant reductions in sensitivity to all noradrenergic effects observed. In extracellular recordings, NE (50 µM) could no longer elicit either long-lasting potentiation of perforant path evoked population potentials or enhance repetitive stimulus-induced Ca^{2+} influx, after kindling. Intracellularly, we observed significant impairment of NE-induced depolarization, blockade of accomodation and the associated AHP, as well as an inability to block Ca^{2+}-dependent regenerative potentials. Furthermore, accomodation of firing and the AHP were, themselves, reduced significantly in slices from kindled rats compared to those from sham-operated controls.

In summary, our results support two main conclusions: (1) NE-induced long-lasting plastic changes in dentate gyrus granule neurons require functional NMDA receptors to be persistently encoded, and (2) large decrements in granule cell sensitivity to NE are associated with kindled epilepsy, a type of neuronal plasticity induced by brief, high-frequency stimulation.

With respect to the first point, it is important to note that the depolarization and R_N increase *during* NE application were not impaired by the NMDA antagonist APV, suggesting that enhanced activation of NMDA receptors is secondary to this effect and only required for long-lasting plasticity to be established. This may result either by bringing the granule cell membrane into a range where voltage-dependent Mg^{2+} blockade of NMDA receptors[16] is relieved and tonically released glutamate now activates NMDA receptors, or, via intracellular cAMP or another second messenger, altering the behavior of the NMDA receptor from the intracellular side. Once such alterations had occurred, enhanced tonic activation of NMDA receptor-mediated Ca^{2+} influx would then trigger long-term plasticity.

In terms of our kindling results, they are potentially significant in context of the role of NE in dentate gyrus long-term plasticity. While in unkindled slices NE is required for full expression of long-term plasticity, a prior history of induction of long-term plasticity renders the dentate gyrus insensitive to either β_1 receptor mediated actions on passive membrane properties, enhancement of repetitive firing or AHP blockade, or α_1 receptor mediated blockade of Ca^{2+} potentials, indicating a general decrease in sensitivity to NE. It may be that, once NMDA receptors are up-regulated, NE can no longer further enhance NMDA receptor activation.

We offer the hypothesis that this may represent a novel protective mechanism against further modification of synaptic efficacy. Such a "write protect" of stored information traces is a requirement if long-term neuronal plasticity induced by high-frequency stimulation is, indeed, a substrate of memory formation. These findings also shed light on the apparent variability of NE-induced plasticity in adult brain and may represent similar protective changes in previously modified synapses. Indeed, in the visual system, modificational sensitivity to NE is lost after a neuronal network has formed its final design[17]. Future studies in the developing brain may find that, prior to the activation of mechanisms protecting against further long-term changes in synaptic strength, NE-induced long-term plasticity, as well as plastic actions of other neuromodulators, are general phenomena. Understanding regulation of such "write protect" mechanisms opens up new approaches to learning disorders and epilepsy in both young and aged brain.

Supported by DFG Grant SFB220-B3 to U.H., Canadian Medical Research Council and I.W. Killam Fellowships to I.M., and an Alexander von Humboldt Foundation Fellowship to P.K.S.

REFERENCES

1. Crow and Wendlandt, Nature 259:42-44,1976.; Mason and Iversen, J. Comp. Physiol. Psychol. 91:165-173,1977.
2. Assaf, et al., J. Physiol. (Lond.) 292:52P,1979.
3. Bliss, et al., J. Physiol. (Lond.) 334:475-491,1983.; Stanton and Sarvey, J. Neurosci. 5:2169-2176,1985.
4. Altman and Corcoran, Brain Res. 270:174-177,1983. McIntyre and Edson, Exp. Neurol. 77:700-704,1982.
5. Neuman and Harley, Brain Res. 273:162-165,1983.; Stanton and Sarvey, Brain Res. 361:276-283,1985.
6. Harris, et al., Brain Res. 323:132-137,1985.; Wigstrom and Gustaffson, Neurosci. Lett. 44:327-332,1984.
7. Peterson, et al., Brain Res. 311:176-180,1984.
8. Stanton and Heinemann, Neurosci. Lett. 67:233-238,1986.; Stanton, et al., J. Neurophysiol., in press.
9. Haas, et al., J. Neurosci. Methods 1:323-325,1979.
10. Heinemann, et al., Exp. Brain Res. 27:237-243,1977.
11. Coordinates: 1.8 mm posterior to Bregma, on the midline and 4.2 mm below the cortical surface.
12. Coordinates: 2.5 mm posterior to Bregma, 3.6 mm lateral to the midline and 7.8 mm below the cortical surface.
13. Racine, Electroenceph. Clin. Neurophysiol. 32:281-294,1972.
14. Goddard, Nature 214:1020-1021,1967.
15. Mody and Heinemann, Nature 326:701-704,1987.
16. Davies and Watkins, Brain Res. 130:364-368,1977.; Mayer, et al., Nature 309:261-263,1984; Nowak, et al., Nature 307:462-465,1984.
17. Pettigrew and Kasamatsu, Nature 271:761-763,1978.

Physiological Plasticity

Physiological plant ec...

The Hippocampus and Classical Conditioning

R. F. THOMPSON

Department of Psychology, Seeley G. Mudd Building, University of Southern California, University Park, Los Angeles, CA 90089, USA

When an animal is trained to perform a discrete behavioral response in aversive classical conditioning, e.g., eyelid closure or limb flexion, pyramidal cells in CA1 - CA3 of the hippocampus develop an extraordinary temporal "model" of the amplitude-time course of the behavioral CR. This "model" -- a pattern of increased frequency of discharge within trials -- can be seen even with an individual pyramidal neuron. The hippocampus models behavioral responses as well as "places in space." The properties of this "plastic response model" share many features with LTP.

The hippocampus plays a critically important role in certain aspects of classical conditioning but is not necessary for the acquisition or retention of the basic learned response. On the other hand, the cerebellum is essential for such learned behavioral responses. Further, lesions of the cerebellum that abolish the learned behavioral response also abolish the hippocampal model in the CS period but not in the US period. Current work focussing on interaction of hippocampus and cerebellum will be considered.

Evidence to date argues strongly that at least some aspects of the training-induced plasticity in hippocampal pyramidal cells are the result of long lasting plastic processes occurring within the hippocampus. This evidence will be reviewed in the context of cellular mechanisms of memory storage and retrieval.

H. L. Haas G. Buzsàki (Eds.)
Synaptic Plasticity in the Hippocampus
© Springer-Verlag Berlin Heidelberg 1988

Long-Term Potentiation: Its Effect on Classically Conditioned Behavior and Hippocampal Network Properties

T. W. Berger, J. R. Balzer, T. P. Harty, G. B. Robinson, and R. J. Sclabassi

Departments of Behavioral Neuroscience, and Neurological Surgery,
University of Pittsburgh, Pittsburgh, PA 15260, USA

Abstract: The possibility is explored that long-term potentiation (LTP) of hippocampal synapses is induced by classical conditioning. LTP of perforant path–dentate synapses is shown to influence the rate of behavioral learning, and to alter functional network properties of the hippocampus. Data relevant to prerequisites for the induction of LTP by conditioning stimuli also are presented.

Classical conditioning of the rabbit nictitating membrane (NM) response using a tone conditioned stimulus (CS) and a corneal airpuff unconditioned stimulus (UCS) is associated with a marked increase in the firing rate of hippocampal pyramidal neurons. The increase develops gradually over the course of training, and occurs with a progressively shorter latency within the CS–UCS interval (Berger et al., 1983). The pattern of pyramidal cell discharge correlates positively with the amplitude-time course of the NM conditioned response (CR), and the onset of this pattern precedes onset of the CR by at least 45–50 msec. These cellular changes are highly dependent on temporal contiguity of the CS and the UCS in the same manner as NM behavior, so they are correlates of associative processes underlying learning.

Several years ago, we noted a number of parallels between the characteristics of LTP and these learning-induced changes in hippocampal activity, such as rapid development, dependence on specific stimulus conditions, small number of stimulations needed for induction, among others (Berger, 1982). Additional parallels came from observations that NM conditioning is associated with a gradual increase in granule cell response to stimulation of the perforant path (Weisz et al., 1984), and an increase in glutamate binding in hippocampus, a phenomenon shared with LTP (Mamounas et al., 1984).

To test further the hypothesis that LTP or an LTP-like phenomenon occurs during NM conditioning, we examined the effect of pretraining LTP on learning rate, and found that animals with LTP induced in perforant path–dentate synapses learned at significantly faster rates than controls (Berger, 1984). We reasoned that LTP had an enhancing effect on acquisition rate because its effects are consistent with the changes in pyramidal cell activity that occur with conditioning. That is, LTP results in simultaneously increased levels of excitability in a large proportion of hippocampal neurons: 60–70% of pyramidal cells exhibit an enhanced response to stimulation after NM conditioning (Berger et al., 1983; Disterhoft et al., 1986).

H. L. Haas   G. Buzsàki (Eds.)
Synaptic Plasticity in the Hippocampus
© Springer-Verlag Berlin Heidelberg 1988

This interpretation was based on LTP's effect on synaptic strength. It is possible that LTP also affects the frequency responsiveness (or, dependence on time since previous activation) of granule cells, and it may be this effect rather than the change in synaptic strength that enhances learning. We tested the effect of LTP on granule cell frequency response using nonlinear systems analytic procedures described elsewhere (Berger et al., in press; Sclabassi et al., in press). Briefly, trains of 4064 electrical impulses with randomly varying inter-impulse intervals (Poisson distribution) were applied to the perforant path. Granule cell output, measured as amplitude of the population spike, was expressed in the form of a functional power series expansion that allows the input-output transformational characteristics of the perforant path-dentate projection to be computed as the terms of the functionals. The terms were computed to the third order, which allowed us to determine the dependence of population spike amplitude on the interval since a previous impulse, and on the intervals since two previous impulses.

This analysis was performed before and after LTP induction in chronically implanted animals. Results showed that in addition to the predicted increase in average amplitude of all population spikes elicited by train stimulation, LTP also significantly reduced the dependence of granule cell response on inter-impulse interval. For example, while inhibition of the population spike still occurred at short intervals of stimulation (e.g., 10-20 ms), virtually no facilitation was seen at longer intervals (e.g., 100 ms). Likewise, LTP virtually abolished third order interactions, or the dependence of granule cell response on intervals of the two preceding impulses.

Further experiments revealed that these effects were not due to saturation, or a post-LTP reduction in frequency modulation because of a maximal response to each impulse. When the stimulation intensity used for random train stimulation was reduced to equalize pre- and post-LTP population spike amplitudes, a marked reduction in the nonlinearity of dentate output still was observed post-LTP. Thus, in a manner which is unrelated to its effect on synaptic strength, LTP leads to a significant reduction in the dependence of granule cell response on the frequency and pattern of input from the entorhinal cortex. Several mechanisms apparently underlie LTP, and these data may represent their integrated consequences at the network level, or may indicate that mechanisms in addition to those responsible for increased synaptic strength are needed to account fully for LTP's effects. These findings also require that any behavioral consequences of LTP be evaluated with respect to its effects on transformational properties of the potentiated pathway, as well as on synaptic potency.

The possibility that an LTP-like phenomenon occurs in response to behavioral conditioning raises the issue of whether afferents to the hippocampus discharge at frequencies or patterns sufficient to induce LTP. Pyramidal neurons within the hippocampal and entorhinal cortices exhibit "complex" spikes, i.e., bursts of action potentials with short interspike intervals representing frequencies of firing very similar to the 100-400 Hz that most efficiently induce LTP experimentally. Neurons of these regions are spontaneously active, however, so that such complex spikes do not occur against a silent background. Moreover, their mean firing rates are much lower than during complex spike discharges. Thus, if bursts of short interspike intervals are sufficient to induce LTP, they will occur within the context of a continuous and variable sequence of action potentials having a low mean rate.

We tested this hypothesis by stimulating the perforant path with trains of electrical impulses having such characteristics. Inter-impulse intervals of each train were determined by Poisson distributions having mean rates of 0.5, 1.0, 2.0, 3.3, 5.0, 6.7, or 10.0 Hz; the corresponding frequency ranges were 0.05-250 Hz, 0.1-500 Hz, 0.2-1K Hz, 0.33-1.5K Hz, 0.5-2.5K Hz, 0.67-3K Hz and 1.0-5K Hz, respectively. Stimulation intensity during train stimulation was constant, but across trains, varied between 10-75% of that necessary to produce maximum spike amplitude.

Stimulus trains with mean frequencies of 0.5-3.3 Hz did not induce LTP, even when high intensities were used. In contrast, frequencies of 5.0-10.0 Hz could induce LTP at low stimulation intensities, with a probability that was positively correlated with mean frequency. Less than 200 total impulses were needed to produce LTP when the mean frequency was 10.0 Hz. Thus, LTP in the dentate gyrus can occur in response to synaptic input that resembles the continuous, variable discharge of entorhinal cortical neurons provided the mean discharge rate is 5.0-10.0 Hz. Because so few impulses are needed to induce LTP at higher mean frequencies, it is possible LTP occurs in response to brief increases in the firing rate of entorhinal neurons, such as might occur in response to conditioning stimuli.

Berger, T.W. (1982) Hippocampal cellular plasticity induced by classical conditioning. Neurosci. Res. Progr. Bull. 20: 723-729.

Berger, T.W. (1984) Long-term potentiation of hippocampal synaptic transmission affects rate of behavioral learning. Science 224: 627-630.

Berger, T.W., Eriksson, J.L., Ciarolla, D.A. & Sclabassi, R.J. (in press) Nonlinear systems analysis of the hippocampal perforant path-dentate system. II. Effects of random train stimulation. J. Neurophysiol.

Berger, T.W., Rinaldi, P., Weisz, D.J. & Thompson, R.F. (1983) Single unit analysis of different hippocampal cell types during classical conditioning of the rabbit nictitating membrane response. J. Neurophysiol. 50: 1197-1219.

Disterhoft, J.F., Coulter, D.A. & Alkon, D.L. (1986) Conditioning causes intrinsic membrane changes of rabbit hippocampal neurons in vitro. Proc. Nat. Acad. Sci., U.S.A. 83: 2733-2737.

Mamounas, L.A., Thompson, R.F., Lynch, G. & Baudry, M. (1984) Classical conditioning of the rabbit eyelid response increases glutamate receptor binding in hippocampal receptor membranes. Proc. Nat. Acad. Sci., U.S.A. 81: 2548-2552.

Sclabassi, R.J., Eriksson, J.L., Port, R.L., Robinson, G.B., & Berger, T.W. (in press) Nonlinear systems analysis of the hippocampal perforant path-dentate system. I. Theoretical and interpretational considerations. <u>J. Neurophysiol.</u>

Weisz, D.J., Clark, G.A. & Thompson, R.F. (1984) Increased responsivity of dentate granule cells during nictitating membrane response conditioning in rabbit. <u>Behav. Brain Res.</u>, <u>12</u>: 145-154.

Neurones of the Medical Temporal Lobes and Recognition Memory

I. P. RICHES, F. A. W. WILSON, and M. W. BROWN

Department of Anatomy, University of Bristol, Bristol BS8 1TD, United Kingdom

Neurones recorded from the monkey medial temporal lobe display evidence of memory for the previous occurrence of visual stimuli. In the inferomedial temporal cortex, 26 (20%) of 128 single units responded more strongly to the first presentations of visual stimuli which had not been seen recently than to subsequent presentations. Such declining responses were also found in the basolateral amygdala and ventral putamen. No such responses were found in the hippocampus, dentate gyrus or subicular cortex. These findings suggest that the inferomedial temporal cortex, rather than the hippocampal formation, plays a central role in recognition memory.

The memory deficits produced by bilateral medial temporal lobe lesions in man and monkey include prominent recognition memory impairments (Mishkin, 1982; Squire, 1986). Subsequent to the lesion, human patients report no familiarity for material presented even a few moments earlier, if their attention has been distracted. The basis of recognition memory is registration of the previous occurrence of stimuli. The reported experiments have examined the change in response of neurones recorded in the medial temporal lobes of behaviourally trained monkeys when presentations of visual stimuli are repeated.

The visual stimuli comprised >500 objects and >50 coloured geometric patterns. These stimuli varied in their familiarity to the monkey; some were seen many times a day, most had been seen only a few times, or never, before. The objects were presented for approximately 2s against a white background. No response was required of the monkey. Trials on which pieces of fruit or a syringe containing fruit juice were presented and given to the monkey were pseudo-randomly interspersed between trials on which objects were shown. (Brown et al. 1987). The geometric patterns were presented for 0.5s on a video monitor as part of a delayed matching to sample task (Brown, 1982). In the delayed matching task a monkey had to press either a right or a left panel to obtain fruit juice reward, dependent on whether two successively presented patterns were the same or different. In this task two stimuli were used over a block of 8-20 trials before being changed. Eye and hand movements were video monitored.

In the inferomedial temporal cortex (peri- and pro-rhinal cortex and areas TE1 and TG), 20%, i.e. 26 of 128, of the recorded units had

H. L. Haas   G. Buzsàki (Eds.)
Synaptic Plasticity in the Hippocampus
© Springer-Verlag Berlin Heidelberg 1988

responses which declined strongly and significantly (paired t-tests, P<0.05) between the first and second presentations of either objects and/or geometric stimuli, if these had not been seen recently. In the basolateral amygdala 2 (10%) of 20 units and in the ventral putamen 2 (7%) of 28 units were similarly responsive. In more lateral parts of inferotemporal cortex (other parts of area TE) 1 (3%) of 34 units responded in that way. However, none (0%) of 268 units recorded in the hippocampus, dentate gyrus or subicular areas nor any (0%) of 82 units in areas TF or TH was found to show such decremental responsiveness.

Of the inferomedial temporal units, 7 were tested to discover whether their responses recovered after intervening presentations of other objects (maximum delay tested >100 sec); for 6 units (86%) the responses did not recover (paired t-test, P<0.05). The responses of one of these units is illustrated. For one of the 10 units whose responses declined following the introduction of new stimuli in the delayed matching task there was sufficient data to show that responses did not recover (paired t-test, P<0.05) after intervening blocks of trials (>60s).

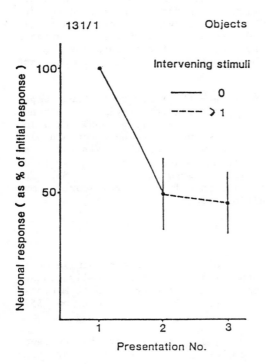

The mean (± S.E.M.) response of a prorhinal unit to repeated presentations of 9 different objects each shown three times. There was one or more intervening presentations of other stimuli between the second and third presentations in each case. Note that the response did not recover to its initial value.

Thus these units displayed evidence of memory for the previous occurrence of stimuli even in the presence of distraction. In some cases this memory lasted for at least many seconds, though the data also indicate that there were units with declining responses for which the memory span was probably less than a minute. Evidence for longer-term information storage was found by comparing the units' responses to stimuli which were unfamiliar to the animal to their responses to familiar objects, to foods and to the juice-containing syringe. For the 21 inferomedial temporal units with declining responses to repeated presentations of objects, the mean firing rate in response to the first presentations of unfamiliar objects was significantly (binomial test, P<0.01) higher than that for familiar objects for 17 (81%) of the units. It was higher than the mean response to the syringe for 18 (86%) of the 21 units and higher than the mean response to food for 20 (95%).

Hence units within the medial temporal lobes display evidence of memory for the previous occurrence of stimuli, but such units were not found within the hippocampal formation. The response decrements are not readily explicable by gross changes in behaviour, arousal, attention or visual fixation. Although unitary response decrements were found in the delayed matching task, behavioural performance did not parallel such decrements. The decremental type of response appears to be an endogenous property of the neurones, rather than one induced by training procedures; its occurrence was incidental to task performance.

These results indicate that whatever the role of the hippocampal formation in memory, it is not in registering the previous occurrence of stimuli. The results do not preclude the hippocampal formation being involved in other aspects of memory, nor it being concerned with more complex aspects of recognition memory such as the registration of contextual (Brown, 1982) or positional (O'Keefe and Nadel, 1978) information, or the choice of behavioural response (Gaffan, 1985). The findings suggest that the adjacent inferomedial temporal cortex may have a central function in recognition memory.

References

Brown, M.W. (1982) Effect of context on the response of single units recorded from the hippocampal region of behaviourally trained monkeys. In C. Ajmone Marsan and H. Matthies. (Eds.), Neuronal Plasticity and Memory Formation, Raven Press, New York, pp. 557-573.

Brown, M.W., Wilson, F.A.W. and Riches, I.P. (1987) Neuronal evidence that inferomedial temporal cortex is more important than hippocampus in certain processes underlying recognition memory. Brain Research, In Press.

Gaffan, D. (1985) Hippocampus: memory, habit and voluntary movement. Phil. Trans. R. Soc. B, 308, 87-99.

Mishkin, M. (1982) A memory system in the monkey. Phil. Trans. R. Soc. B. 298, 85-95.

O'Keefe, J. and Nadel, L. (1978) The hippocampus as a cognitive map. Clarendon Press, Oxford.

Squire, L.R. (1986) Mechanisms of memory, Science, 232, 1612-1619.

This work was supported by the MRC.

Hippocampal Involvement in Rabbit Eyeblink Conditioning

J. F. DISTERHOFT, H. R. READ, and E. AKASE

Department of Cell Biology and Anatomy, Northwestern University Medical School, Chicago, IL 60611, USA

A conditioning-specific reduction in the afterhyperpolarization (AHP) response has previously been demonstrated in CA1 pyramidal cells in hippocampal slices from well conditioned rabbits. The present studies compare slices taken from groups of rabbits which had received the same number of eyeblink training trials. Since the AHP was reduced only in the rabbits which learned, these data show definitively that the AHP reduction is dependent upon behavioral acquisition. In another set of lesion-behavior studies, we have begun exploring the contribution hippocampus makes even in short-delay blink conditioning. We have found that extinction occurs considerably faster in hippocampectomized rabbits.

INTRODUCTION

Neurons in the hippocampus demonstrate substantial involvement in the acquisition and retention of simple associative tasks in mammals, as evidenced by their enhanced firing to conditioned and unconditioned stimuli during learning (1, 2). In fact, CA1 and CA3 pyramidal neurons show a striking "neural model" of the conditioned blink response in well trained rabbits (3). We have begun investigating the cellular basis of this enhanced excitability with biophysical analyses of CA1 pyramidal cells in brain slices from well trained rabbits. A series of experiments done in collaboration with D. Coulter and D. Alkon demonstrated a conditioning-specific reduction in the amplitude and time course of the afterhyperpolarization (AHP) in these cells (4,5). The AHP is a manifestation of a Ca^{++}-mediated outward K^+ current and is one brake on action potential rate in vivo (6,7). The fact that the alteration was seen in brain slices, separated from their normal afferent and efferent connections, indicated that this alteration was local to hippocampus. This reduction was present even in the absence of synaptic transmission, substantiating the postsynaptic nature of this change (8). Thus we have suggested that a reduction in the AHP is one postsynaptic cellular alteration, local to hippocampus, which underlies the enhanced excitability pyramidal neurons demonstrate after associative learning in the intact animal.

The studies briefly summarized here address two points. First, our previous work had concentrated on animals that were well trained. We wished to demonstrate a relationship between behavioral acquisition and AHP size in rabbits which had received the same amount of training but acquired the response to different degrees (9). Second, previous lesion experiments have demonstrated no effect of hippocampal removal on acquisition or retention of short-delay blink conditioning (10,11). But

H. L. Haas   G. Buzsàki (Eds.)
Synaptic Plasticity in the Hippocampus
© Springer-Verlag Berlin Heidelberg 1988

hippocampus appears to be primarily involved in transferring information from the short- to long-term memory store, so its removal may have a maximal effect on a learned response still in the process of consolidation. We tested this proposition for extinction of the short-delay blink response (12).

METHODS and RESULTS

In the acquisition study (9), rabbits were blink conditioned for two 80 trial sessions. A short-delay paradigm was used in which the tone conditioned stimulus (CS) overlapped and coterminated with the periorbital shock unconditioned stimulus (US). Intracellular recordings were made from hippocampal CA1 pyramidal neurons within brain slices prepared 24 hours following the second training session. The rabbits were separated into two groups on behavioral criteria. The High group (N=10) showed an average of 94% blink CRs on the second training day, the Low group (N=6) 4.4% CRs (p<.01). Biophysical recordings from CA1 pyramidal neurons in brain slices prepared from the two groups showed a marked difference in the AHP recorded after 4 action potentials elicited by intracellular current injection. The mean AHP amplitudes in the High group (N=18) was -3.0±.36 mv, that in the Low group was -4.0±.37 mv (p<.05). These AHP differences were present in the absence of High-Low group differences in mean action potential height (88 vs. 87 mv), resting potential (-67 vs. -68 mv) and input resistance (64 vs. 70 Mohms).

Lesioned rabbits underwent bilateral suction lesions of the dorsal hippocampus. Rabbits were trained in the short-delay paradigm to a behavioral criterion of two successive 10-trial blocks with 8 or more CRs. After 24 hours, extinction was begun. The major difference between the lesioned (N=11) and intact (N=9) animals in the first 40 extinction trials was that hippocampectomized rabbits showed faster extinction than did the controls (20 vs. 49% CRs, p<.025). Ongoing experiments are enlarging the groups and adding neocortical lesion control animals to the study.

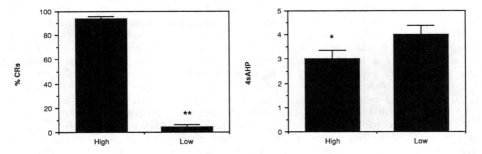

Fig. 1. High and Low group behavioral acquisition and AHP amplitude compared.

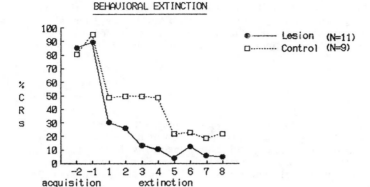

Fig. 2.   Blink CRs shown by intact and hippocampectomized rabbits.

COMMENTS

We have previously demonstrated a conditioning-specific reduction in the AHP in well conditioned rabbits (1,2).   In the experiments summarized here, all rabbits received the same number of training trials.   Those rabbits which learned had CA1 pyramidal cells with significantly reduced AHP amplitude and duration (Fig. 1).   The group which did not acquire the conditioned response showed mean AHP amplitudes comparable to the Naive group in our previous study (5).   These data definitively link the AHP reductions to behavioral response acquisition.   In addition, they demonstrate that the AHP is not reduced merely as a side effect of paired CS-US trials.

Our lesion/behavior study (Fig. 2) further demonstrates that hippocampus makes a contribution to memory storage of even simple associatively learned tasks. The lesioned animals we have studied showed faster extinction in simple short-delay eyeblink conditioning.   Our observations are in contrast to previous reports which have demonstrated no effect of hippocampal removal on extinction of nictitating membrane/eyeblink conditioning in the short-delay paradigm (10,11).   It appears that testing retention of a learned response still in the process of consolidation is more sensitive to the role of hippocampus in laying down the conditioned reflex arc. Previous studies   have tested completely trained rabbits, perhaps thereby involving   brainstem/cerebellar   circuitry   (13).

The studies summarized here, in combination with our previous work (4,5,8), show that hippocampal pyramidal neurons undergo localized biophysical alterations during associative learning.   The reduced AHP is a postsynaptic alteration likely to be a major contributor to the enhanced cellular excitability observed   as animals learn the tone-puff association. Finally, with appropriate behavioral evaluation, the hippocampal contribution to even simple associative learning tasks is demonstrable after lesions.   Our ongoing experiments are exploring information storage mechanisms during learning at the cellular and molecular level.

REFERENCES

1. Berger, T.W., Clark, G.A. and Thompson, R.F. (1980) Physiol. Psychol. 8, 155-167.
2. Segal, M. (1973) J. Neurophysiol. 36, 840-854.
3. Berger, T.W., Rinaldi, P.C., Weiss, D.J. and Thompson, R.F. J. Neurophysiol. 50, 1197-1219.
4. Disterhoft, J.F., Coulter, D.A. and Alkon, D.L. (1986) Proc. Natl. Acad. Sci. USA 83, 2733-2737.
5. Coulter, D.A., Kubota, M., Moore, J.W., Disterhoft, J.F. and Alkon, D.L. (1985) Soc. Neurosci. Abst. 11, 891.
6. Hotson, J.R. and Prince, D.A. (1980) J. Neurophysiol. 43, 409-419.
7. Lancaster, B. and Adams, P.R. (1986) J. Neurophysiol. 55, 1268-1282.
8. Coulter, D.A., Disterhoft, J.F. and Alkon, D.L. (1986) Soc. Neurosci. Abst. 12, 181.
9. Disterhoft, J.F., Golden, D., Read, H., Coulter, D.A., and Alkon, D.L. (1986) Soc. Neurosci. Abst. 12, 180.
10. Schmaltz. L.W. and Theios, J. (1972) J. Comp. Physiol. Psychol. 79, 328-333.
11. Solomon, P.R. and Moore, J.W. (1975) J. Comp. Physiol. Psychol. 89, 1192-1203.
12. Akase, E. and Disterhoft, J.F. (1987) Soc. Neurosci. Abst. 13, In Press.
13. Thompson, R.F. (1986) Science 233, 941-947.

Human Hippocampal Neuronal Firing to Specific Individual Words and Faces

E. Halgren[1], G. Heit[2], and M. E. Smith[3]

[1]Brain Research Institute and Department of Psychiatry, University of California at Los Angeles, Epilepsy Center, Wadsworth Veterans Administration Medical Center, Los Angeles CA, USA, and INSERM U97, 2 ter, rue d'Alesia, 75014 Paris, France
[2]Brain Research Institute, University of California at Los Angeles and Stanford University School of Medicine, Stanford, CA 95403, USA
[3]INSERM U97, 2 ter, rue d'Alesia, 75014 Paris, France

Recently, we found that some human hippocampal formation units fire specifically to particular words or faces. In this presentation, we will briefly describe this phenomenon (for further details, please see Heit et al., under revision). We then discuss the implications of this finding for how the brain encodes complex cognitive stimuli, and for the physiological mechanism whereby the hippocampus contributes to Recent Memory in humans.

Complex partial epilepsy resistant to medication can be treated successfully with depth electrode identification of epileptogenic tissues and subsequent surgical resection (1). Based on clinical criteria, patients in this study had bilateral depth electrodes implanted in the hippocampus, parahippocampal gyrus, and basolateral amygdala. Action potentials were recorded from immobile insulated 40 micrometer wires for offline correlation with behavioral and physiological events. Common abstract words were visually presented for 0.3 seconds every 2.5 seconds. Following the input block, in which the subject was instructed to memorize each of 20 words, 8 blocks of recognition testing occurred. The same 10 words from the initial 20 were repeated in each block intermixed with 10 words (nonrepeats) that only occurred once in all eight blocks. Thus each repeated word occurred a total of 9 times. During the 8 recognition blocks the subject was instructed to keypress to repeated words. Each unit had a sum histogram formed from its response to all 9 presentations of each of the repeated words. All 10 histograms for a unit were then visually compared to each other for preferential responses to one of the repeated words. The null hypothesis of a unit having equal levels of excitation to all repeated words was statistically tested using a randomization technique.

Thirty of 39 units tested had visually and statistically significant evidence (p < .01) of preferential responses to one repeated word. Of the 39 units tested with words, 14 were also tested during recognition memory with photographs of strangers' faces. Two units, both located in the left anterior hippocampus preferentially responded to one of the repeating faces. All 30 responsive units had increased firing to their preferred stimulus that began 300-500 msec after stimulus onset and lasted 200-500 msec. In contrast, visual sensory responses in the human MTL are concentrated in the posterior hippocampal formation and have latencies less than 100 msec. Furthermore, when tested, the units described here did not respond to a reversing checkerboard pattern. Units with word specificity were observed regardless of whether or not a behavioral response was made

H. L. Haas   G. Buzsàki (Eds.)
Synaptic Plasticity in the Hippocampus
© Springer-Verlag Berlin Heidelberg 1988

to that word. Thus, the stimulus specific responses were not directly related to simple visual features or to keypress.

What is the significance of this specific firing to only one word out of the ten repeating words? Have we found the legendary 'grandmother cell'? (a la Konorski)--the cell whose firing is specific to an exquisite combination of features extracted by sensory and sensory association cortices, and unique to a specific very highly complex and meaningful stimulus? Certainly, cells that fire to one word, but not to 9 others have a highly abstract firing correlate. The occurrence of such cells in 3 structures with very different internal wiring schemes suggests that they indeed may be fairly common. However, the cells we found clearly deviate from those predicted by the grandmother legend in several critical points. First, the lexical representation of a word (as reflected by vocabulary size or word/nonword discrimination) is not affected by human hippocampal lesions. Thus, the hippocampal word-specific cells are not necessary for neurally encoding words. In fact, studies of eye-fixation during reading suggests that lexical access is far advanced prior to the 300 msec onset latency of the hippocampal word-specific cells. This, of course, is consistent with neuroanatomy--Wernicke's area in humans appears to be homologous to the parieto-temporal association cortex area that projects to the hippocampus in monkeys. Furthermore, simple considerations of sampling (we recorded from few cells and few words yet found many word-specific cells) clearly imply that the same cells should be found to fire to other words in a different context, and, conversely, that many hippocampal cells are simultaneously firing to the same word. Thus, the hippocampal word-specific firing appears not to represent the one neuron that encodes only one word, but a group of neurons that fire to a particular word in a particular context.

How might this contextually word-specific firing contribute to a function that the hippocampus is required for: contextual recognition? Psychological studies have identified the retrieval of the previous context of presentation as being critical for recognition of word repetition. Basic hippocampal anatomy and physiology are consistent with word-specific firing helping to link the word to its previous context, and thus aiding in contextual retrieval (2). The first time a word is presented, it would be decoded by Wernicke's area (and related cortex), and projected to the hippocampus together with firing defining the context. The hippocampal formation projects back to association cortex, and thus would participate in cortico-hippocampal-cortical activity pattern defining the event (=word-in-context). The cortico-hippocampal synapses and hippocampo-hippocampal synapses participating in this loop could be strengthened by LTP, so that when the word is re-presented, the previous context may be evoked by the hippocampo-cortical projection.*

----

* The same mechanism would support the hippocampal contribution to recall of recent events. In contextual recognition, the event (word in this case) is given, and the context retrieved; in contextual recall, the context is given, and the event is retrieved. Note also that, in this model, LTP functions to stabilize information representation. This may be distinguished from an LTP function of causing the hippocampus to fire more strongly to a repeated stimulus, allowing familiarity to be detected as strong hippocampal output. In fact, we have seen no overall differences in hippocampal firing to repeated versus nonrepeated stimuli.

Independent support for this model comes from a consideration of the timing of the word-specific units with respect to the field-potential components evoked in the same task (3). Within the hippocampus, two such components have been observed, peaking at 460 ('N4') and 620 ('P3') msec after word onset (4). These components have been examined at the scalp in normal subjects in a large number of tasks, where it appears that the N4 represents post-lexical associative activation to meaningful stimuli in a meaningful context, and the P3 represents closure of processing. In this particular contextual word recognition task, the N4 declines with word repetition, whereas the P3 grows larger. This appears to directly reflect the effect of contextual-retrieval in making the word-context relationship evolve more rapidly and surely. If, as suggested above, the word-specific units in the hippocampus are contributing to contextual retrieval, then they should fire at the time when the N4/P3 to repeated words begins to diverge from the N4/P3 to nonrepeated words. This, in fact, is what is observed. Furthermore, when the dominant hippocampal formation (together with overlying structures) is removed surgically to relieve seizures, repetition no longer has an effect on the N4/P3 to words! Thus, the contextually word-specific units appear to be in the right place, at the right time, and with the right firing-correlates, to make the contribution assigned to them in this model.

These studies are preliminary crude beginnings. The precise 'cognitive fields' of the word-specific units remain to be determined (e.g., will a cell firing to a particular word fire to the same word in another modality, or to a synonym?). It is also unknown whether word-specific units are indeed influenced by the context of presentation. Of greater importance for a neurobiological theory of human memory, the animal homologues of these human phenomena need to be established. The similarity of the specific-word units to the rat place cells is obvious. Other human hippocampal cells have been observed to fire during 'voluntary movement,' for example, during the keypress in the contextual word-recognition task. These bear a clear resemblance to theta cells in the rat hippocampus, and perhaps to the rabbit hippocampal cells that fire to conditioned stimuli. The N4/P3 field-potential sequence bears no relationship to movement. However, its dominant frequency of about 6 Hz suggests that it could be homologous to a single cycle of the 'cholinergic' theta, emitted to interesting stimuli. In the highly visual human presented with a brief visual stimulus, a single cycle of information acquisition/association/integration (i.e., of gestalt formation and closure) might suffice, whereas for the perambulating rat primarily using touch and olfaction, several successive cycles may be more appropriate.

1. A.V. Delgado-Escueta and G.O.Walsh, Neurology 35, 143-154 (1985).
2. E. Halgren in The Neuropsychology of Memory, N. Butters and L. Squires, eds. (Guilford, New York, N.Y. 1984) pp.165-181.
3. E. Halgren and M.E. Smith, Human Neurobiology, in press (1987).
4. M.E. Smith, J.M. Stapleton, E. Halgren, Electroencephalgr. Clin. Neurophysiol. 63, 145-159 (1986).

The Induction of Long-Term Synaptic Plasticity in the Dentate Gyrus Is Modulated by Behavioral State

C. R. Bramham and B. Srebro

Department of Physiology, University of Bergen, Årstadveien 19, 5000 Bergen, Norway

SUMMARY   Freely moving rats received high-frequency stimulation of the perforant path-granule cell pathway during slow-wave sleep (SWS) and during a still-alert (SAL) behavioral state. Trains given in SAL induced LTP of the dentate population spike height, spike onset latency, and the epsp-spike relation more often than did trains delivered in SWS. In some cases tetanization in SWS was followed by a long-term depression (LTD) of these field potential measures. The results suggest that the ability of hippocampal neurons to undergo long-term synaptic plasticity is dynamically modified according to the behavioral state of the animal.

Studies in freely moving rats have shown that the efficacy of neuronal transmission in the major hippocampal pathways changes with the behavioral state of the animal (1). We investigated the possibility that the ability of neurons to sustain long-term potentiation (LTP) of the perforant path-granule cell system is also modulated by behavioral state.

Seventeen male Sprague-Dawley rats were anesthetized and electrodes cemented in position to allow chronic stimulation of the perforant pathway with recording of evoked potentials and EEG from the dentate hilus. Experiments were begun at least one week after surgery in environmentally habituated animals and were performed between 8 A.M. and 1 P.M. Standard field potential measurements were collected in a still-alert state (SAL), slow-wave sleep (SWS), and during rapid eye movement sleep (REM), as defined by behavioral and EEG criteria. On the first 3 days of testing, stimuli were delivered during SAL at regular intervals throughout the experimental period to detect possible fluctuations in the response, and data for input-output (I-O) curves were collected in SAL and SWS to establish the behavioral modulation pattern of the field potential. On Day 4 animals received a high-frequency stimulus train (400 hz, 20 ms, 8 sequences with at least a 10 s rest interval) during either SAL or SWS. A second train was given on the next day (after the response returned to the baseline level) in the other behavioral state. Since the epsp is larger in SAL compared to SWS the current intensity used during the second tetanization was adjusted to evoke an epsp equivalent to that of the first train. Seven of these rats were later tetanized during REM sleep. The position of the recording electrode was verified histologically in 5 animals.

H. L. Haas   G. Buzsàki (Eds.)
Synaptic Plasticity in the Hippocampus
© Springer-Verlag Berlin Heidelberg 1988

EXPERIMENTAL PROTOCOL

Day 1, 2 and 3	Day 4	Day 5	Day 6 or 7
Stability test I-O Curve	Stability test I-O Curve	Stability test I-O Curve	Stability test I-O Curve
	Train 1 in SWS or SAL	Train 2 in other state	Train 3 in REM

The criterion for long-term changes of each field potential measure was a significant difference between values obtained before and between 10 to 90 minutes after tetanization (t-test correlated samples; p<0.05). This statistic gave percentage criteria for the response change of about ± 10%, for the population spike height, epsp slope, and epsp- spike relation, and ± 3% for the spike onset latency.

The main result of this study is summarized in Table I.

TABLE I. BEHAVIORAL STATE AND THE INDUCTION OF LONG-TERM SYNAPTIC PLASTICITY IN THE DENTATE GYRUS

Number of cases

	Spike height*		EPSP slope		Spike latency*		EPSP-Spike*	
	SWS	SAL	SWS	SAL	SWS	SAL	SWS	SAL
LTP	8	14	7	10	2	11	7	12
LTD	3	0	1	1	7	2	5	1
N.C.	6	1	8	4	7	2	4	2

* The effects of high-frequency stimulation given during SAL and SWS were significantly different (Chi-Square >5.99, df=2, p<0.05, except for epsp-spike where p<0.1). N.C. - no change.

LTP of the spike height, spike onset latency, and epsp-spike relation occurred more often when trains were delivered during the SAL state (range 60-95% of cases), as compared to SWS (range 5-45% of cases). In fact, in several animals there was a depression of these measures after tetanization in SWS. The direction of the epsp changes for the SAL and SWS groups, however, was not significantly different (p>0.1). In addition, repeated collection of input-output curves confirmed the pattern of behavioral modulation of field potentials (SWS vs SAL) described by others (1). This pattern did not change after tetanization.

The magnitude and direction of the field potential changes for 3 individual animals are illustrated in Fig. 1 (page 3). LTP of the spike height and onset latency was consistently seen after high-frequency stimulation in SAL, while the same procedure in SWS produced no change or even LTD. Interestingly, animals subsequently tetanized during REM sleep (7 cases) showed changes similar to those following the SAL train. Finally, in animals which demonstrated LTP, there was no group difference between SWS and SAL in the magnitude of increase of any field potential measure (t-test independent samples p>0.1).

The results suggest that the capacity to sustain long-term synaptic plasticity is not a fixed, static property of hippocampal neurons but is dynamically modified according to the behavioral state of the animal. Further investigation of the mechanism and possible functional significance of this phenomenon could be rewarding.

1.   Winson, J., and Abzug, C.J., Neurophysiol., 41 (1978) 716-732.

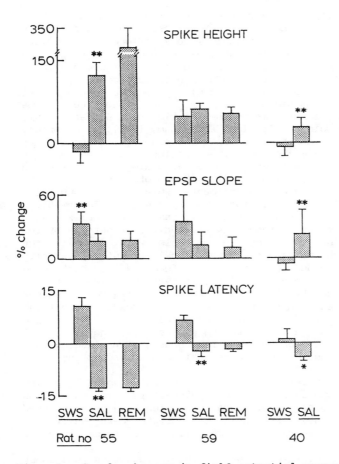

Fig. 1. Sample changes in field potential measures after tetanization in differet behavioral states. Histograms show means ± S.E.M. (of 4 responses) collected at 6 time points between 10 and 90 min post-train. Significant differences between SWS and SAL on the basis of a t-test for correlated samples are marked (**p<0.05; *p<0.1). Changes following tetanization in REM are included for comparison.

Parallel Studies on Learning and LTP in the Dentate Gyrus

S. LaRoche, O. Bergis, V. Doyere, and V. Bloch

Départment de Psychophysiologie, C.N.R.S. and Université de Paris XI,
91190 Gif-sur-Yvette, France

The concept of network remodelling after increased activity as a basic mechanism for the storage of neural representations forms a framework on which most physiological models of memory are built. Long-term potentiation of synaptic transmission in the hippocampus, an example of activity-dependent strengthening of synaptic connexions, has therefore attracted much attention as a plausible candidate for a physiological mechanism subserving mnemonic processes. The original assumption became strengthened as more was known about the characteristics, properties and mechanisms of LTP (e.g. Goddard, 1981; McNaughton, 1983; Voronin, 1983; Bliss and Lynch, 1987). As examples, the induction process, durability, and the cooperative/associative property of LTP, are all in the stream of the predictions one may formulate if LTP is to be viewed as a neural analog of learning. In addition, LTP is accompanied by the kind of biochemical and morphological changes at synaptic elements which have long been proposed as potential sustrates for the storage of information. However, the trace of an event, the engram, cannot be localized at a particular synapse but is rather distributed throughout the brain, synaptic reorganization occuring in multiple relays within the relevant network (Bloch and Laroche, 1984). Indeed synaptic plasticity is not in itself a model of memory, but a functional property upon which memorizing activity could, at least in part, be based. Parallel studies on learning and LTP thus foster a search for a neural change at a focused locus assumed to be part of a widespread, hypothetical network through which the information is encoded and retreived upon reexcitation. It follows that the question addressed is whether LTP at a selected node within the network may represent a valuable candidate for a mechanism upon which synaptic connexions are strenghtened as a result of a learning experience.

Although no single experiment has yet unequivoqually proven the link between LTP and learning, the hypothesis received converging support from diverse behavioural paradigms which have been reviewed recently (Laroche, 1985). We shall concentrate here on recent observations from our laboratory which illustrate three different strategies of investigation.

We have used classical conditioning in rats to a tone-shock association which results in the tone suppressing lever-pressing for food, because of the very large behavioural literature which permits description of the learning processes underlying response change under a well defined conceptual framework (e.g. Dickinson, 1980) and because it allows cellular analysis of brain substrates of learning in a behaving animal. Tone-shock association in rats produces a large

H.L. Haas   G. Buzsàki (Eds.)
Synaptic Plasticity in the Hippocampus
© Springer-Verlag Berlin Heidelberg 1988

increase in the frequency of hippocampal cell discharges to the CS which occurs after a very few pairings (Olds et al., 1972; Bloch and Laroche, 1981). This associative neural response is seen in the hippocampus and the dentate gyrus, but not in the entorhinal cortex (Laroche, Falcou and Bloch, 1983), can last for at least two months (unpublished data), and represents a neural index of the acquired CS-US associative representation (Laroche, Neuenschwander-El Massioui, Edeline and Dutrieux, 1987). This suggests that hippocampal circuits are a branch of a network engaged in the processing of at least some aspect of the association.

After associative learning, we examined the amount of LTP in the dentate gyrus to brief tetani on perforant path fibers (Laroche, Bergis and Bloch, 1983). LTP was induced by 10 high-frequency (400 Hz) short duration (20 msec) stimulus trains (5-min intertrain interval), delivered to the perforant path two days after the last of 6 tone-shock conditioning sessions. As compared to pseudoconditioning, learning the tone-shock association resulted in an increased LTP at perforant path-granule cell synapses. In addition, when conditioning at both the behavioural and cellular levels was facilitated by a posttrial stimulation of the reticular formation, this LTP strengthening effect was further enhanced. The same results were obtained after discriminative conditioning. These data suggest that the development of associative changes in the dentate gyrus is accompanied by lasting changes in synaptic function. Since artificially-induced LTP benefits from conditioning, it might be inferred that both processes share, at least in part, common underlying synaptic mechanism(s).

A second series of experiments was designed to examine whether biochemical indices of presynaptic changes associated with LTP are similarly associated with conditioning. LTP in the dentate gyrus is accompanied by an increase in the release of both endogenous and prelabelled glutamate (see Bliss, Douglas, Errington and Lynch, 1986; and Lynch et al., this volume), and it has been proposed by the authors that the maintenance of LTP can be in part explained by the sustained increase in transmitter release from tetanized pathways. We examined the $\underline{in\ vitro}$ release of preloaded, radiolabelled glutamate and aspartate in the dentate gyrus and areas CA1 and CA3 of the hippocampus taken from rats previously trained in a tone-shock classical conditioning paradigm (Laroche, Errington, Lynch and Bliss, 1987). One hour after the last of 4 conditioning sessions, the dentate gyrus and subfields CA3, CA1 of the hippocampus were removed bilaterally, and slices prepared for subsequent $\underline{in\ vitro}$ analysis of K^+-stimulated, Ca^{2+}-dependent release of (^3H)-glutamate.

Potassium-stimulated, Ca^{2+}-dependent release of glutamate was significantly greater in slices of dentate gyrus and area CA1 prepared from conditioned animals than from pseudoconditioned animals. The increased release of glutamate following conditioning establishes a similarity between LTP and associative learning. Further, this finding identifies a biochemical change which may underlie the lasting changes in synaptic function built up during learning.

Finally, a third strategy of investigation was developed in which electrical stimulation of the perforant path served as a conditioned stimulus in a conditioned suppression paradigm. This approach allows direct estimation of the strength of a population of synapses necessarily involved in the learning task. When a high-frequency stimulation of the perforant path (400Hz-20msec trains at 1 Hz during 6 sec), with an intensity set to a value which gave a population spike of about 1 mV, was used as CS, the animals displayed LTP of both the population EPSP and population spike and learned the brain stimulation-shock association. Animals however failed to learn when the CS intensity was below spike threshold and consequently LTP not produced. In an another group, each perforant path tetanizing stimulus, above spike threshold, was preceded by a high-frequency stimulation of the contralateral hilus (400Hz-20msec, 8 msec interval onset to onset). In some animals, LTP of perforant path-granule cell synapses was blocked by the commissural trains while in others LTP was only masked during the first conditioning session and developed thereafter. Learning was significantly retarded in this group and a significant positive correlation was found between the magnitude of LTP reached after conditioning and the behavioural conditioned response to perforant path test trials. These data demonstrate that perforant path trains can be used as a CS in a conditioned suppression paradigm when stimulation parameters allow LTP to develop at the activated synapses. The parallel postponement in LTP and behavioural conditioning when nearly concomitant commissural and perforant path trains are used further suggests a correlation between increased synaptic strength and learning the CS-US association.

In conclusion, the data obtained under these three strategies of investigation provide converging experimental evidence that an LTP-like phenomenon occurs during learning. This mechanism may selectively strengthen the activated synapses during learning and could presumably account for the specification of the relevant network by experience in the process of active/inactive memory shifting (Bloch and Laroche, 1984). Future direction of research will further address the question of the degree of similarity between LTP and learning-induced changes in synaptic function as well as that of both the nature of the inductive signal and the kinetics of this process.

References

Bliss, T.V.P., Douglas, R.M., Errington, M.L. & Lynch, M.A. (1986) J. Physiol. (london), 377:391.
Bliss, T.V.P. & Lynch, M.A. (1987) In: Long-term Potentiation: Mechanisms and Key Issues, Eds. P.W. Landfield, S. Deadwyler, Alan R. Liss, NY.
Bloch, V. & Laroche, S. (1981) Behav. Brain Res., 3:23.
Bloch, V. & Laroche, S. (1984) In: Neurobiology of Learning and Memory, Eds. G. Lynch, J.L. McGaugh, N.M. Weinberger, Guilford, NY.
Dickinson, A. (1980) Contemporary Animal Learning Theory, Cambridge Univ. Press, Cambridge.
Goddard, G.V. (1981) In: Brain and Behaviour, Advances in Physiological Sciences, Eds. G. Adam, I. Meszaros, E.I. Banyai, Peryanom, Akademiai Kiado, Budapest.
Laroche, S. (1985) In: Brain Plasticity, Learning and Memory, Advances in Behavioural Biology, Vol. 28, Eds. B.E. Will, P. Schmitt, J.C. Dalrymple-Alford, Plenum, NY.
Laroche, S., Bergis, O.E. & Bloch, V. (1983) Neurosci. Abstr., 9:645.
Laroche, S., Errington, M.L., Lynch, M.A. & Bliss, T.V.P. (1987) Behav. Brain Res., 25:23.
Laroche, S., Falcou, R. & Bloch, V. (1983) Behav. Brain Res., 9:381.

Laroche, S., Neuenschwander-El Massioui, N., Edeline, J.M. & Dutrieux, G. (1987) Bevav. Neural Biol., 47:356.

McNaughton, B.L. (1983) In: Molecular, Cellular and Behavioural Neurobiology of hippocampus, Ed. W. Siefert, Academic, NY.

Olds, J., Disterhoft, J.F., Segal, M., Kornblith, C.L. & Hirsh, R. (1972) J. Neurophysiol., 35:202.

Voronin, L.L. (1983) Neurosci., 10:1051.

Subject Index

DATE DUE

DEC 1 - 1989

JUL 2 9 1995

JUN 1 3 1997

APR 1 6 2003

JUL 0 9 2017

SEP 1 1 2017

DEMCO NO. 38-298